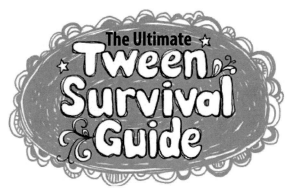

Eating Disorders

Understanding Them, Preventing Them, and Helping a Loved One

By Dina Zeckhausen, PhD

Illustrated by Julia Mahood

This book is dedicated to:

Addie, Ethan, Olivia, Marcella, Emmy, John John, Jordan, and Maddie.

Thank you for sharing your experiences & advice to help other kids.

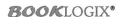

Alpharetta, Georgia

Copyright © 2012 by Dina Zeckhausen

2964 Peachtree Road, Suite 324 • Atlanta GA 30305

www.dinazeckhausen.com

www.tweensurvivalguide.com

ISBN: 978-1-61005-237-5

Library of Congress Control Number: 2012918974

Printed in the United States of America

This paper meets the requirements of ANSI/NISO Z39.48-1992 (Permanence of Paper)

This book is not intended as a substitute for the medical advice of physicians. The reader should consult a physician regularly in any matters relating to his/her health, particularly with respect to any symptoms or illness that may require diagnosis or medical attention.

Cover Art and Illustrations: Julia Mahood

All quotes taken from BrainyQuotes.com

TABLE OF CONTENTS

When Someone You Love Has an Eating Disorder

How to use the Ultimate Tween Survival Guide to Eating Disorders

My name is Dina Zeckhausen. I'm a psychologist and a mom. I've been helping people recover from eating disorders for over twenty years. I discovered something important: an eating disorder doesn't just affect the person suffering with it. An eating disorder impacts the lives of everyone who loves that person. It is extremely stressful and confusing for loved ones to understand what is happening and know how to help. I also discovered there were plenty of books for parents of kids and teens with eating disorders, but there were no books for kids from age eight to thirteen. Sadly, these days more tweens have friends, siblings and even parents who have eating disorders.

As a tween who wants to learn more about eating disorders, this book is for YOU!

Are you curious to learn more about eating disorders? Are you wanting to know how NOT to get one? Are you worried about someone you know who is struggling with an eating disorder?

Then this book was written for YOU.

Because more females than males struggle with eating disorders, throughout the book I'll refer to your loved one as "she." Of course, if your friend, sibling or parent is a male, the information still applies to him!

I hope this book feels like an honest conversation with a wise aunt who'll give you straight answers to tough questions. I'll chat with you like you're an intelligent person who wants to make smart decisions.

This book has three parts.

In Part One you'll meet ED, the nickname we give an Eating Disorder. You'll learn some Key Words and find out why eating disorders are such a problem for so many people these days.

Part Two will tell you everything you need to know to avoid getting an eating disorder and to have a healthy mind and body!

Part Three will give you lots of helpful information and advice if someone you love has an eating disorder.

Finally, I'll answer Frequently Asked Questions from tweens just like you!

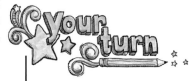

Look for this graphic to indicate a Your Turn section. These are places for you to jot down your thoughts, take fun quizzes, cut out awesome quotes, make a pledge, share your feelings and sketch your ideas. The more time you spend on the Your Turn sections, the more you'll learn and the better you'll feel!

Part 1

Understanding Eating Disorders

Meet ED

When someone has an eating disorder, they have a voice in their head that sounds like a bully. Often when people are in the process of recovering from their eating disorder, they give this inner voice a name. Some call it "ED" (for Eating Disorder).

When this person does something kind, ED says,

> You're Selfish deep inside!

When this person does something well, ED says,

> You could've done better!

When this person looks in the mirror, ED criticizes her body. ED says,

> You're a FAT PIG!

(Even if she is thin.)

Even though many people love her, ED says,

> They don't really know you. If they did, they wouldn't love you!

ED always forces this person to compete with everyone around her, and the competition that ED really wants to win is the **Thinnest Person Contest.** (I'll bet you didn't even know there was a contest going on!)

Another thing about ED: like a shape-shifting monster, ED may look different in different people. Sometimes ED even changes form in the same person. ED can force a person to starve one moment and then force that same person to eat a ton of food. I'll tell you more about all the forms that ED can take in a few pages.

The other super-annoying thing about ED is that he loves numbers. He is obsessed with them!

He's like a calculator with no "Off" button, constantly adding and subtracting numbers: calories, pounds, fat grams, pants sizes. Give ED a number and he'll make a judgment about it: too fat, too big, too much. Imagine going through each day with this judgmental, critical, numbers-obsessed bully inside of your head. ED makes it hard to be happy, relaxed, or feel okay.

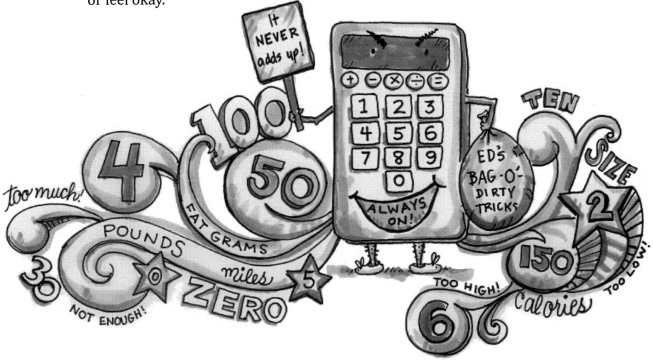

Key Words For You To Know

Self-esteem

Self-esteem is how you think of yourself as a person. It's like having an inner voice that watches what you do and tells you if you're lovable and good enough. If you have positive self-esteem, you generally think of yourself, deep down, as a good, nice, and worthwhile person. You have an inner voice that sounds like a BFF. It encourages you with thoughts like *Great job!* or *You're a nice person* or *You look good today!* That voice also forgives you when you mess up. *It's OKAY. Nobody's perfect. What did you learn so you can do better next time?* If you have negative self-esteem, that voice in your head is very hard on you, especially if you do something that you don't feel good about. It criticizes you and kicks you when you're down. *You're a stupid idiot! You're a bad person.* When your inner voice is negative and harsh most of the time, it's like having a bully inside your brain. Having already met ED, you can guess the type of self-esteem of someone with an eating disorder.

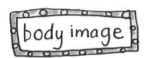 body image

Body image is about how you view your body, and how you feel about what you see (lots more about this on Page 50). *While self-esteem is about who you are on the inside, body image is about how you look on the outside.* This may sound weird, but body image is not necessarily about how you *actually* look. A person with an eating disorder has an extremely negative body image, meaning they do not like the way their body looks. Whether they are fat, average-sized, thin or dangerously skinny, they tend to see their bodies as humongous. When there is a big difference between how a person views their body and how it actually looks, it's called a *distorted body image.* Ever look at yourself in one of those distorting fun-house mirrors at the fair? You can go from ridiculously huge to scary skinny just by moving to the right or left. What makes it so funny is knowing that what you see is not real. But imagine if you saw a distorted image of yourself every time you looked in the mirror. This would not be hilarious at all.

Scientists are studying the brain to figure out exactly why someone with an eating disorder cannot see their own body accurately. They think it may be because her brain is not getting proper nourishment from enough of the right foods. The part of the brain that perceives the body isn't working right because it is starving!

It can be very frustrating to tell someone she's beautiful, while knowing that she just doesn't believe you. She would like to believe you, but ED won't let her.

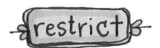

To restrict something means to take it away. Ever have a friend who got in trouble and was *on restriction?* That means the things they love—watching TV, talking on the phone, hanging out with friends—were taken away as punishment. When someone restricts their food, it's like being on restriction, only the thing that gets taken away is food. A person who restricts their food for too long may develop an eating disorder known as anorexia.

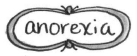

A person with anorexia has restricted her food so much that she loses enough weight that it can hurt her body. Now, you may be thinking, *Wait a minute. I thought losing weight was a good thing! Everyone in America is trying to lose weight!* But when someone loses too much weight, it can actually be harmful to their mind and their body.

Ways that Restricting Harms the Mind of a Person with Anorexia:

- All she thinks about is food, so she can't concentrate on the normal things in daily life.

- She may be spacey and forgetful.

- She may be grumpy, moody, and short-tempered.

Ways that Restricting Harms the Body of a Person with Anorexia:

- She may feel weak and tired because her body doesn't have enough fuel (food) to run properly.

- Her hair can become dry and fall out; her nails can become weak and breakable.

- Over time, poor nutrition can weaken her bones, causing them to fracture easily.

- Eventually lack of nutrients can damage muscles and organs, including the heart and brain.

- Years later when she's ready to have kids, she may have trouble getting pregnant because starvation causes hormonal problems.

So if she feels so yucky all the time, why won't she just eat?

When a person has anorexia, even though her tummy may be growling and all she can think about is food, ED will not let her eat enough of the right foods. ED might only let her eat certain foods that he has decided are safe. ED will come up with weird food rules: "You may eat grapes and lettuce, but you may not eat cheese or ice cream!" or "You can only eat breakfast if you have exercised for ninety minutes" or "You can only eat at noon and six o'clock but you may not eat after seven o'clock."

Even though ED thinks he is an expert on food and nutrition, he is actually quite wrong about what a body truly needs to be healthy. ED will say, "OKAY, maybe everyone else needs protein, carbohydrates, and fat in their diets, but you do not! You must live on less food than other normal humans because if you eat like everyone else, you will become fat!"

Because of this voice in her head, a person with anorexia becomes addicted to the feeling of hunger. The hungrier she is, the happier ED is. This may seem weird and hard to imagine. So even if you baked your loved one the most delicious tasty chocolate brownie in the universe, presented it to her on a pretty plate with roses all around it, ED would not let her eat it.

When she is super hungry but she says no to delicious food, ED says,

When she has eaten and her tummy is full, ED says,

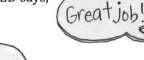

ED is a jerk, huh?

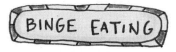

BINGE EATING

The opposite of restricting food is to binge on food. When a person binges they eat a lot of food all at once, way past when their tummy says, "Stop!" Have you ever eaten past full? We all do this sometimes, especially on holidays that involve lots of yummy food like Thanksgiving and Halloween. When you do this, your tummy hurts, you get in a bad mood and you probably want to lie around because you have no energy. A person who binge eats a lot has an eating disorder known as binge eating disorder.

BINGE EATING DISORDER

People with binge eating disorder (BED for short) are good at hiding their binge eating. You may rarely see them binge because they feel so embarrassed about it. They usually only do it when they're alone. Binge eating feels scary and out of control. If someone does this often and over a long period of time, they can gain an unhealthy amount of weight.

Usually people with binge eating disorder got this way because they went through a time of restricting their food through dieting or anorexia. After a while, their hungry tummies finally said, "Enough! I'm too hungry! I can't take it anymore!" They discovered, to their horror, that once they started eating they couldn't stop.

You can imagine this feels very scary and out of control. People with binge eating disorder have that same nasty ED voice in their heads, always telling them what failures they are because they eat too much. Binge eating disorder harms the mind and the body.

Ways that Binge Eating Harms the Mind of the Person with BED:

- She has low self-esteem because ED is constantly saying, "You are fat and out of control!"

- She feels like she has a shameful secret that she must hide from everyone she loves.

- She thinks about food all the time, has trouble concentrating, and feels grumpy.

Ways that Binge Eating Harms the Body of the Person with BED:

- Overeating can lead to weight gain which can cause back and knee problems, heart problems, and other health issues.

- The stress of being overweight in our society (which is constantly pressuring people to be thin) can actually add to the physical damage of being overweight.

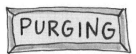

Sometimes a person feels so yucky and guilty about eating (especially if she has eaten too much) that she *purges*. To *purge* means to get rid of something. When someone cleans out their closet and gives away old clothes, they say they have purged their closet. This feels great! When someone wants to get rid of the food in her stomach fast, she may make herself throw up. A person who binges and then purges has an eating disorder known as bulimia.

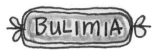

As you know, everything you eat will leave your body within a few hours when you go to the bathroom. But a person with bulimia cannot wait; she wants that food out *now*. It's hard to imagine making yourself throw up on purpose since vomiting is one of life's worst feelings! But remember how mean ED gets when a person feels full or fat? "You are fat, bad and disgusting!" he says. The misery that ED causes from feeling too full is actually a *worse* feeling than throwing up. Yes, it's that bad.

Purging a lot can be quite harmful to the mind and body.

Ways that Purging Harms the Mind of a Person with Bulimia:

- Her self-esteem goes way down because she is secretly doing something that she finds disgusting.

- She feels like she has to hide and lie to people she loves, and that feels awful!

- She feels grumpy, thinks about food all the time and has trouble concentrating.

Ways that Purging Harms the Body of a Person with Bulimia:

- The stomach acid coming up her throat can hurt the lining of her throat.

- The stomach acid can damage her teeth.

- Losing fluid and electrolytes (important substances in your gut) can cause damage to muscles and organs.

This is why you should *never* try to get rid of the food in your stomach by throwing up. EXCEPTION: If you are choking or you have a stomach flu or you ate something poisonous by accident, then throwing up is okay.

over-exercising

You've heard a million times that exercise is healthy and good for you, and it is. But if you do too much of anything, even a good thing, you can turn it into a bad thing. Sometimes people with eating disorders over-exercise to try to lose weight or change the way their body looks. Over-exercising can damage the body's joints, bones and organs. How much is too much? Some examples might be:

- If she takes a day off from exercise she will be in a terrible mood.

- She puts exercise before everything else.

- She exercises even when the weather is bad or it might not be safe.

- She exercises even if she is sick or injured.

If you do too much of anything, even a good thing, you can turn it into a bad thing.

RECOVERY

Recovery is the word that describes the process of getting better from an eating disorder. You may have heard this word referring to the flu or another illness. Your loved one can recover from her eating disorder by getting help from experts. Recovery involves listening to her body's signals so that she does not restrict, binge, over-exercise or purge. Because she may have stopped listening to her body a long time ago, it may take months or years for her to hear and respond to those signals again. It may seem odd to think that your loved one needs to learn something as simple and basic as eating right. It almost seems as crazy as learning to breathe or sleep! But our relationship with food is so complicated that it can be tough to get things back where they should have been all along.

Recovery also means that your loved one will be able to argue with ED, and win! While it's impossible to make the voice of ED disappear completely, it is possible to make ED's voice quieter and less powerful.

One woman who recovered from an eating disorder described it like this: "When I was in the middle of my eating disorder, the sound of ED was as loud as standing next to a car with the alarm going off. Now that I am recovered, I hear the sound of ED, but it's like an ambulance far off in the distance."

Now that you've met ED and learned some key words, you may be wondering how ED came to be such a powerful force inside of so many perfectly good brains! Here's the back story...

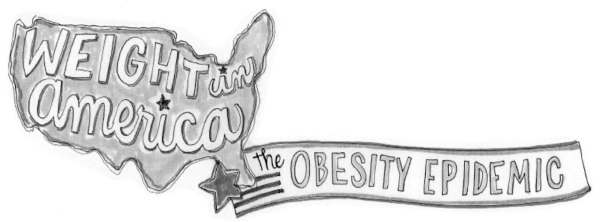

It's no wonder there are so many people struggling with their weight. These days there's more food around than ever before, we spend hours in front of our computers, TVs and X-Boxes, and we eat whenever we feel stressed, bored, or upset. The media likes to call this problem "The Obesity Epidemic." So people created a diet industry, figuring that they could make money helping Americans lose weight. And they have certainly succeeded in making money! American's spend fifty billion dollars (that's billion with a "b") every year on diet books, diet pills, and diet foods. So, has the diet industry helped America become healthier, fitter or thinner? No!

In fact, our obsession with diets has only made the situation worse. Ever watch *The Biggest Loser* on TV? Did you know that many of those contestants gain back all of their weight after the show is over? Extreme dieting and over-exercising are impossible to maintain for an entire lifetime. Not only are there more fat Americans than ever before, now there are millions of people like your loved one who are battling eating disorders that started as an innocent little diet.

Not only are there more fat Americans than ever before, now there are millions of people like your loved one who are battling eating disorders that started as an innocent little diet.

Eating, sleeping, and breathing are three of our most basic human survival activities. Because our bodies require food, sleep, and oxygen to stay alive, they force us to eat, sleep and breathe whether we want to or not! Think about it: do you think you could just decide to go a few nights in a row without sleeping? Do you think you could just decide to go a few hours without breathing? Pretty ridiculous, huh?

And yet it seems that everyone in America thinks they should be able to resist their powerful urge to eat. This insane activity is called "going on a diet."

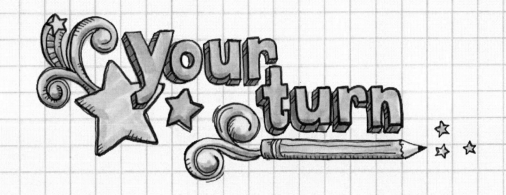

write about how you would feel if you went a Long time...

    without breathing:

    without sleeping:

    without eating:

Media Images

At the same time that Americans are gaining weight, the images of bodies that we see in the media are getting smaller! Think about the bodies of the people that you see in magazines, on TV, in movies, on billboards and in video games. Most of the females are ridiculously thin and many have large breasts. Often they are dressed in sexy clothes that show off their bodies. Images of men include big muscles and "six-pack abs." It's natural to compare your body to those bodies. Does it seem like the world is plotting to make you feel bad about yourself?

To fight this ridiculousness, you must understand a couple of key points:

 Images in the media are not real. There is a popular computer program called Photoshop (you may even know how to use this!) that changes the images you see. You've probably played around with different software programs that change, distort, or perfect your picture on a computer screen. These days, cameras can get rid of wrinkles and make your teeth whiter before you even upload the picture! **Every image that you see in the media has been altered.** Legs, arms, necks, and bodies are changed to look longer and thinner. Wrinkles, pores, and pimples are made to disappear! Therefore, comparing your body to a media image is like comparing yourself to a cartoon, which I assume you are too smart to ever do!

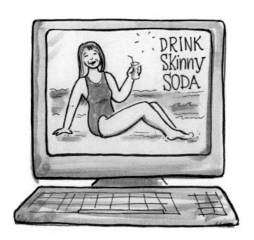 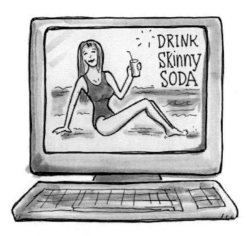

Before Photoshop...   *...and after!*

Many models and actresses are not healthy. Eating disorders are common in the entertainment industry where entertainers are pressured to be extremely thin. They often starve themselves, purge, over-exercise—all of the behaviors we discussed in the eating disorder section—in order to look extremely thin for the cameras. Do not envy them! That part of their lives may be miserable.

 Advertisers are trying to make you feel insecure; this is how they make money! Here's the logic: You see a picture of a teenage girl's perfect, flawless (Photoshopped) face or body in a magazine. You look in the mirror and feel bad because you are not perfect. You think *Maybe if I buy that cream/lotion/ diet product then I will look like that girl!* So you save up your money and buy something. Meanwhile, the company that made you feel bad has your money and you have a product that will never make you look like the person in the magazine. You see the trap?

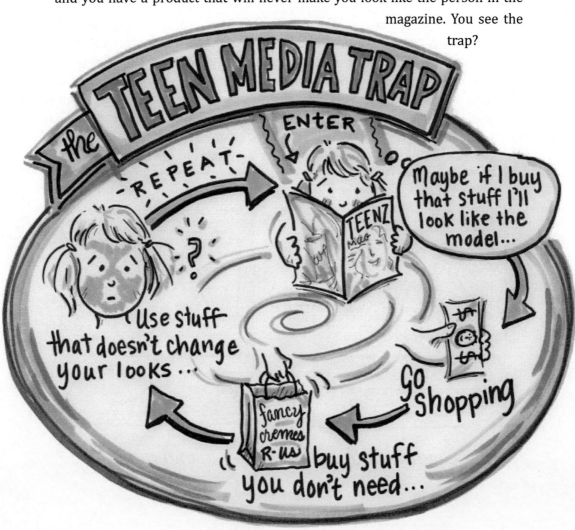

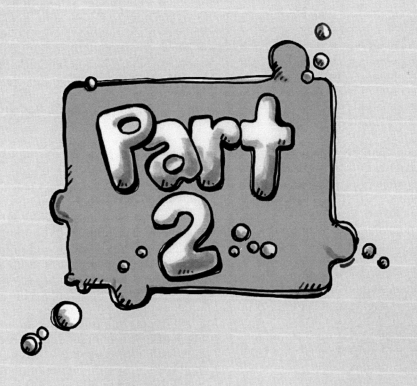

Avoiding Eating Disorders and Taking Care of You!

As you discovered in Part 1, many people today are unhappy with their bodies, struggling with their weight and going on diets. All this may make you confused about how YOU should be eating. Part 2 will help you stay in touch with the wisdom of your body and show you how to take care of yourself so you don't end up with an ED in your head!

Normal Eating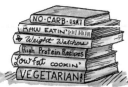

There are so many different ways to eat, it's hard to know what's normal. Here are some helpful guidelines for figuring out what in the world it means to be a normal eater.

When You Eat

Experts in nutrition recommend eating every three to four hours (except while you're sleeping, of course). That means eating breakfast, a mid-morning snack, lunch, a mid-afternoon snack, dinner, and maybe a little something before bed. You're probably thinking that sounds like a lot of food. It's actually better for your brain and your body to eat smaller amounts of food throughout the day than to eat three huge meals. If you don't spread out your food throughout the day you may end up starving in the evening because you didn't eat enough that day.

I realize that, as a kid, you don't always have control over when you eat. Sometimes you're tummy is screaming, "Hungry!" but you don't get lunch for two more class periods. If you know it's going to be a long time before you eat again, try to plan ahead: eat a bit more breakfast to hold you over, or take a snack to school.

How Much You Eat

The best way to determine how much to eat is to listen to the signals coming from your stomach. A normal eater knows and trusts these signals and uses them as a guide for knowing when to eat and when to stop. Even when your taste buds are screaming for you to keep eating because it tastes good, a normal eater can tell her taste buds, "I know it's yummy, but you can have more later. If you eat too much, you won't feel good."

The problem is that sometimes there are signals around you that are louder than your stomach. Picture yourself at a Mexican restaurant with your friends. The music is loud; you smell the sizzling hot fajitas flying past your table; your friends are talking like crazy and you are digging into that basket of crispy chips and spicy salsa. You love this food, and with everything going on around you it's nearly impossible to listen to your stomach. Even though you are filling up with chips and salsa, you order a meal and just keep eating because noises drown whispers coming from your belly: "I'm full. You can stop eating now." Is it any wonder most people leave a Mexican restaurant feeling not just full, not just stuffed, but sick?

*Become a **Belly Whisperer:** Listen to the quiet whispers of your tummy and you will know the exact moment when it's time to stop eating.*

What You Eat

Every single food falls into one of three categories: Carbohydrates (or Carbs), Protein and Fats. One diet will tell you "Carbs are Evil!" Another will say "Fat is Bad!" But your body needs all three types of food every day to be healthy and function properly. Here's why your body needs them and the best ways to get them!

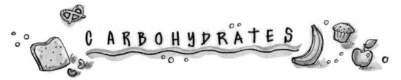

Why do I need them?

- They are your body's main source of energy.
- They are stored in your muscles to give you energy between meals and snacks.
- They are an important source of vitamins and iron.
- They help you feel full.

Some great ways to get your carbs!

- Whole wheat grains: breads, pastas, brown rice, bagels, muffins
- Starchy vegetables: corn, peas, potatoes
- Legumes/beans: pinto beans, black beans, black-eyed peas
- Fruits and veggies
- Pretzels, popcorn, wheat crackers

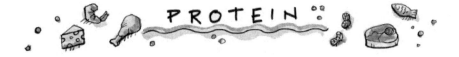

Why do I need it?

- It builds and repairs muscles after exercise.
- It is the building block of major organs.
- It provides a feeling of fullness.

Some great ways to get your protein!

- Lean beef, pork, turkey, chicken, lamb, seafood and fish

- Tofu and veggie burgers, peanut butter and nuts

- Eggs, milk, yogurt, or cottage cheese

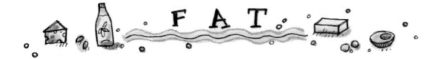

Why do I need it?

- Fat is an important source of energy and helps to maintain the system that fights infections.

- It helps manufacture important hormones.

- It keeps your hair and your nails strong.

- It helps your brain function properly.

- It adds pleasure and deliciousness to foods!

Some great ways to get your fat!

- Peanut butter and other nut butters

- Olive oil, safflower oil, sunflower oil, peanut oil

- Cheese, avocados, olives, nuts and seeds

While it's good for your body to eat mostly healthy food, it's important to allow yourself to eat lots of different types of foods (even "bad" foods!) over the course of a day or a week. It's fine to eat a slice of pie at Thanksgiving, or enjoy cake at the birthday party, or grab a hot dog at the baseball game. Fun foods are an important part of a happy life. If you usually eat fairly healthy food and have an active lifestyle, then you don't need to worry about having occasional treats.

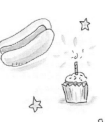

Since you probably don't have your driver's license, you can't exactly hop in the car and buy your own food. Therefore, you don't always get to decide what you're going to eat. However, you still have opportunities to make a choice. You may be starting to notice how different foods affect your body. Some foods give you lots of energy that lasts a long time. Other foods give you a stomach ache. Still others end up making you feel grumpy and sleepy! As you become more aware of how your body works, you can start to pick foods not just for the taste, but also for how they make you feel.

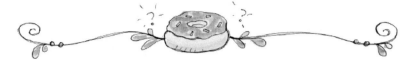

Let's say you have a soccer game on a Saturday morning. Your parents stop at Donuts-R-Us for breakfast. You LOVE donuts, but you've noticed that about an hour after eating a donut you feel tired and grumpy (this is called an energy crash). Since you want lots of energy for your game, it's smarter to have a bagel with cream cheese or peanut butter. The carbohydrates in the bagel and the protein in the cream cheese/peanut butter will give you a long-lasting dose of energy, without an energy crash. If you are curious about how certain foods affect your body, learn more at www.eatright.org.

Why You Eat & Why You Stop Eating

The best reason to eat is that you are hungry. If you listen to your body, you'll have that feeling several times a day. The best reason to stop is that your stomach is satisfied or pleasantly full.

However, sometimes you have to eat even when you aren't hungry just because you may not have a choice in the matter. It may be that this is your only chance to eat for a few hours. Unfortunately, life does not always present us with the perfect food at the exact moment that your body wants it (wouldn't that be nice?) For that reason, normal eating also means being flexible!

It's also normal to eat a little cake just because it's someone's birthday (even if you aren't really hungry). It's normal to get some ice cream because you are celebrating the end of the soccer season. It's normal to eat a couple of cookies when you feel sad. It's normal and okay to do this sometimes. It becomes a problem when you turn to food whenever you feel stressed, bored, sad or excited. Food should just be one of lots of ways that you experience pleasure or help yourself feel better. (You'll discover more about this in the next section.)

How You Feel About Eating

It's very important that you not get mad at yourself about your eating! Normal eating is not perfect eating. If you say mean things to yourself about the way you are eating ("You eat too much. You eat like a pig.") then you might stop listening to your body and instead start paying too much attention to the voice in your head. Remember the key to normal eating is listening to your body!

Why Diets Aren't Cool

When I say "diet," I mean a food plan that tells you when, what, and how much to eat. Most diets recommend avoiding fats, proteins or carbohydrates that our bodies actually need in order to function properly. Many diets force you to write down everything you eat, weigh your food, count calories, add up fat grams or sugar grams or carbohydrate grams. If this sounds like a lot of work, you're right! Imagine constantly doing one terribly long and boring math problem all day, every day. Welcome to Diet Land!

Most people who lose weight on a diet will gain it all back (and more) eventually. You should avoid dieting because it's no fun and it doesn't work.

Plus, there are two dangerous places that a diet can take you:

1. When you are super hungry, and you finally DO get to eat, you may eat way too much, way too fast! Remember the binge we talked about on Page 12? This can occur after a period of not eating enough on a diet. A binge can lead to a purge, and then you are heading down the path to bulimia, which is dangerous and awful!

2. The other danger from dieting, as weird as this sounds, is that you could become addicted to not eating. Remember when we talked about Anorexia on Page 11? Well, it starts with restricting your food and it can quickly take on a life of its own. The danger is that depriving yourself of food might feel so good (and eating can feel so bad) you may not be able to stop once you start, which is also dangerous and awful.

I'm sorry. I hope I didn't freak you out. It's important for you to know the inside scoop about how eating disorders start. Going on a diet is like sending a formal invitation to ED, saying, "Hey, there's a room open in my brain. Got no place to live? Come on in!" I'd rather you be prepared in case he ever shows up at your brain, uninvited. If you hear ED knocking, you'll recognize him and say, "Look, ED, there's no way I'm letting you hurt me. Hit the road!"

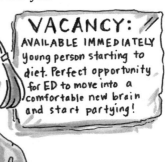

VACANCY: AVAILABLE IMMEDIATELY
Young person starting to diet. Perfect opportunity for ED to move into a comfortable new brain and start partying!

The Goal: Healthy, Not Skinny

Did you know that between ages eleven and fourteen, it is perfectly normal for girls to gain fifteen to twenty pounds? During puberty, boys will gain thirty to forty pounds! Did you know it's also perfectly normal for girls to have their growth spurt one to two years before the boys? So, please don't freak out about this normal weight gain; you're also gaining height! If you remain calm, it will all even out.

The bottom line: it's more important to be healthy and happy than to try to be thin. There are skinny people who smoke cigarettes and don't exercise. There are large people who eat well and are physically fit.

So here's the plan for these next few years...and the rest of your life:

1. Listen to and try to obey your body's Hunger and Fullness signals.

2. Eat mostly healthy foods along with some special treats.

3. Be active every day, whether chasing your dog, dancing in the kitchen or playing a sport.

4. Love and accept your body—whatever size it ends up—when you do 1 – 3.

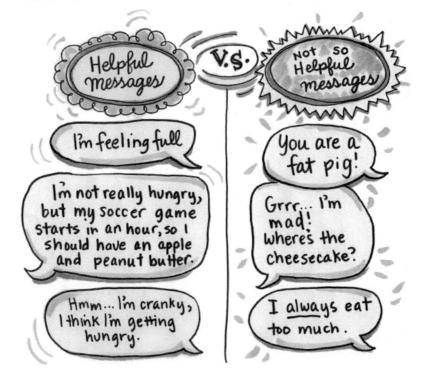

Sports & Pressure About Weight

Participating in sports is a terrific way to get fit and healthy, make great friends, learn important life lessons and have fun!

However, certain sports can actually set the stage for vulnerable tweens and teens to develop eating disorders. Sometimes coaches in cross-country running, gymnastics, ballet, figure skating, or cheerleading may pressure their athletes to lose weight. While it's essential to fuel your body well, it's important to be the healthiest weight for your body type, age, height, and genetics. If you watch the Olympics, you'll notice that the best athletes in the world come in all shapes and sizes. Beware of the message that Thinner is Better!

Even if you are not feeling pressured by a coach, spending hours in a tight leotard in front of a full length mirror surrounded by other girls puts a lot of focus on your body! Compare that to a sport like soccer or softball, where everyone is wearing loose clothing and running around outside. Sports with a strong emphasis on weight and body size can cause negative body image, which leads to unhealthy attempts at weight control.

Sports with a strong emphasis on weight and body size can cause negative body image that leads to unhealthy attempts at weight control.

And this is not just a girl problem! Sports like wrestling, football, and rowing actually have weight categories and different rules for kids based on their size. Some coaches pressure wrestlers to lose weight in order to drop into a lower weight category, believing it's better to be the heaviest guy in a weight class than the lightest. Some wrestlers starve themselves before a weigh-in, then binge afterwards, creating a pattern that can set them up for an eating disorder.

Bottom line:

If you are feeling intense pressure in a sport or from a coach to lose weight and this is making you uncomfortable, speak with your parents or the school counselor. They can help you decide if there might be a sport, coach or team that is a healthier match for you.

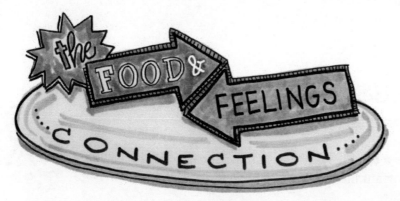

The Food & Feelings Connection

There is complicated relationship between food and feelings. People with eating disorders get their heart signals and their stomach signals mixed up. We're going to help you understand the food-feeling relationship so you won't have trouble in this area. Here's why it gets confusing:

- Sometimes when you're really hungry, you feel grumpy and tearful.
- Sometimes when you're tired, your body says you're hungry.
- Sometimes when you're sad, you want to eat—even if you're not hungry.
- Sometimes when you're anxious, you can't eat even if you are hungry!

I'm going to describe some different situations that kids encounter. Your job is to figure out the best way to handle each food-feeling situation. You may wonder: "Why is it so important to understand the food and feelings connection?" It's so you will:

- Have a healthy relationship with food.
- Weigh what your body is supposed to weigh.
- Be good at taking care of yourself.

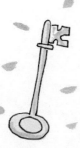

The key is to figure out:

1. What you really feel.

2. What you really need.

3. The smartest action to take that matches up the feeling with the need.

Now, meet Samantha, Andrew, Brendon and Ashley.
Let's see if you can help them make the connection!

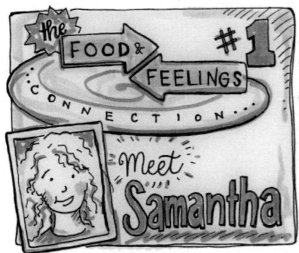

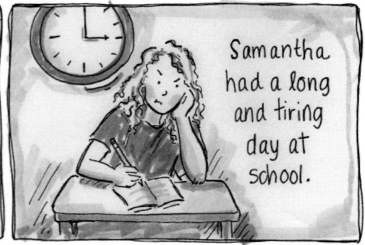

Samantha had a long and tiring day at school.

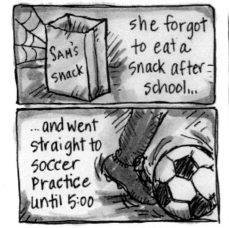

she forgot to eat a snack after school...

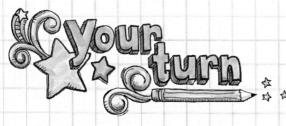

...and went straight to soccer practice until 5:00

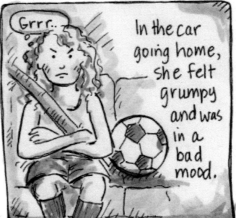

In the car going home, she felt grumpy and was in a bad mood.

She was even yelling at the traffic (which was usually something only her father would do).

1. What did Samantha really feel?

2. What did Samantha really need?

3. What was the smartest action that Samantha could take to match up the feeling and the need?

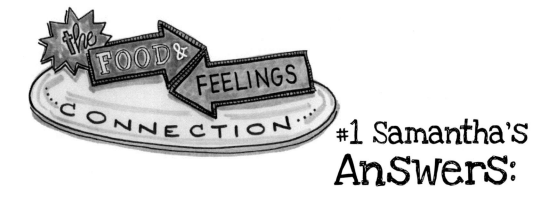

#1 Samantha's Answers:

1. Even though it seemed like Samantha was angry, in fact she was really hungry.

2. She needed to eat. It had been over five hours since lunch.

3. The smartest action was to get some food as soon as possible. When she got home, her mom realized that Samantha was starving. She fixed her an apple with peanut butter. Within a few minutes, Samantha was in a much better mood.

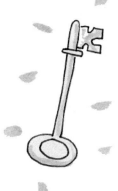

KEY POINT FOR YOU:

Sometimes parents realize when you're upset that you may actually be hungry. It's normal for kids to get so busy that they forget to eat. If that's the case, then eating will help you feel better and happier.

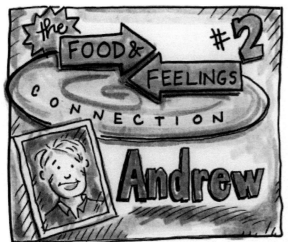

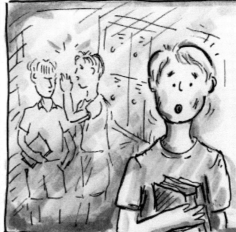

Sam told their friends that Andrew was a loser and then he didn't invite Andrew to his sleepover party. Andrew was surprised, hurt and upset.

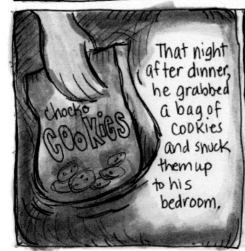

That night after dinner, he grabbed a bag of cookies and snuck them up to his bedroom,

chocko COOKIES

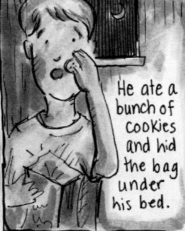

He ate a bunch of cookies and hid the bag under his bed.

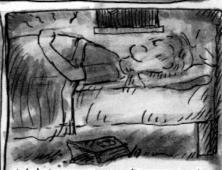

While he was eating the cookies, he felt a little better, but afterwards he felt sick to his stomach. He stopped thinking about his problems but he couldn't ignore his belly ache.

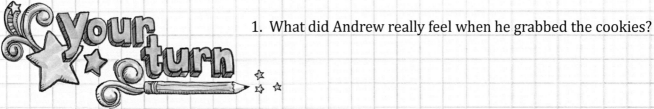

1. What did Andrew really feel when he grabbed the cookies?

2. What did Andrew really need?

3. What was the smartest action that Andrew could take to match up the feeling and the need?

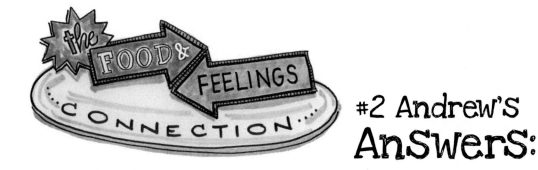

#2 Andrew's Answers:

1. Andrew was really feeling sad, hurt and upset, not hungry.

2. Andrew really needed some comfort and help solving the Sam problem.

3. The smartest action would have been to go to his mom for a hug, and then talk to her about the best way to deal with Sam. That would have actually made him feel better!

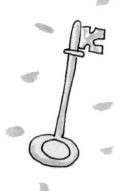

KEY POINT FOR YOU:

By eating food to feel better (when you are not actually hungry!) you are not matching up the Feeling with the Need. Eating to make bad feelings go away not only leaves your first problem unsolved, but adds a second problem: a stomach ache!

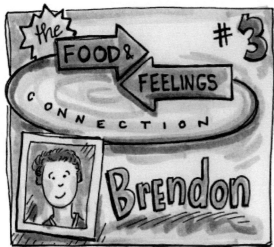
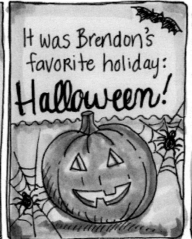
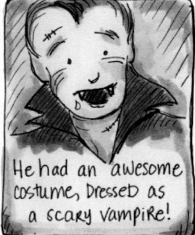
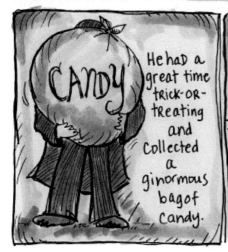
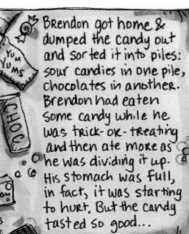
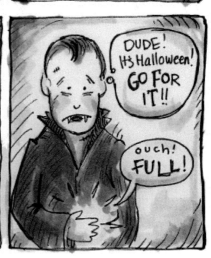

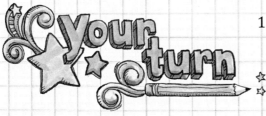

1. What did Brendon really feel?

2. What did Brendon really need?

3. What was the smartest action that Brendon could take to match up the feeling and the need?

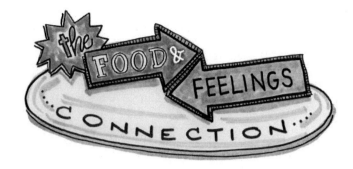

#3 Brendon's Answers:

1. Brendon was feeling full. In fact, he felt so stuffed that his stomach was hurting.

2. He really needed to listen to his tummy instead of his taste buds.

3. The smartest action was to stop eating and put the candy away for later. That way he'd also get to enjoy it over a longer period of time.

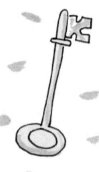

KEY POINT FOR YOU:

If you ignore your stomach when it says "Full" (even if your taste buds are screaming "Go for it!") then you will not feel good. If you do this over and over again, you may end up weighing more than your body wants to weigh, which may mean you'll be unhappy and unhealthy.

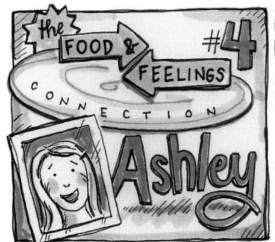

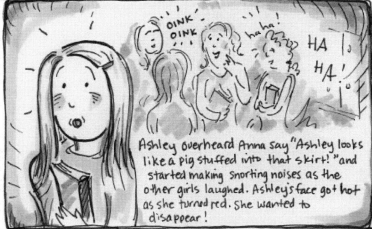

Ashley overheard Anna say "Ashley looks like a pig stuffed into that skirt!" and started making snorting noises as the other girls laughed. Ashley's face got hot as she turned red. She wanted to disappear!

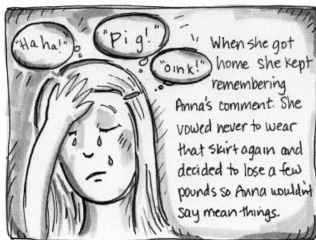

When she got home she kept remembering Anna's comment. She vowed never to wear that skirt again and decided to lose a few pounds so Anna wouldn't say mean things.

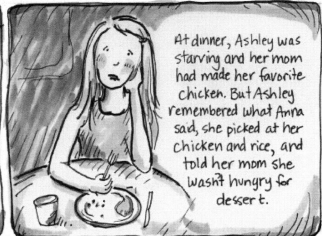

At dinner, Ashley was starving and her mom had made her favorite chicken. But Ashley remembered what Anna said, she picked at her chicken and rice, and told her mom she wasn't hungry for dessert.

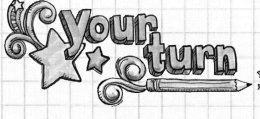

1. What did Ashley really feel?

2. What did Ashley really need?

3. What was the smartest action that Ashley could take to match up the feeling and the need?

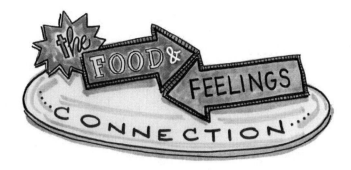

#4 Ashley's Answers:

1. Ashley felt hurt, sad, and embarrassed. She also felt hungry.

2. She needed to feed her body; plus, she needed comfort and help solving the Anna problem.

3. The smartest action was to eat dinner and share the story with a parent who could hug her and help her decide how best to handle Anna—whether to ignore her, confront her, or tell the teacher at school.

KEY POINT FOR YOU:

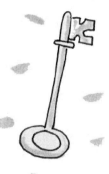

Losing weight will not stop bullies from being mean. Get adult help if you and your buddies can't get the bullies to stop. Starving will only make you weak and could lead to an eating disorder. Feeding your body will help you be confident enough to ignore the mean kids or strong enough to face them head on!

BOREDOM

The Problem

You are a part of the first generation of humans who've grown up with continuous entertainment. Back when your parents were kids, there was radio and there was TV. That was it. There was usually one television set in the house with three channels on it. Everyone in the family watched it together for a couple of hours in the evening. The kids watched cartoons on Saturday mornings. Many families had strict rules against watching TV during the daytime, so kids found ways to entertain themselves. This typically involved running around the neighborhood, making up games, reading books or bugging our siblings.

Today most teens, tweens, and kids have instant access to non-stop technology, whether it's a game on your cell phone, an ipad app, a DS, or an Xbox. While these technologies can be super fun and entertaining, there is a downside.

1. They are addictive. *Technological entertainment gives us Instant Pleasure, but we can quickly become bored with it so we need ANOTHER game and another...and more and more and more.*

2. They are passive. *Technological entertainment does not require much effort from your brain. Over time you can lose the ability to entertain yourself without a screen in front of you. The ability to use your imagination starts to disappear, like a muscle that's never used.*

Because of their addiction to technological entertainment, young people have trouble knowing what to do when they have a moment of free time. They are easily bored and do not know what to do with themselves. So they may turn to the next easiest thing: *eating or not eating.* When I speak to groups of kids, teens or adults and I ask, "Who has ever used food or dieting to deal with boredom?" 95% of the hands in the room go up (maybe the other 5% didn't hear the question). Here's how the logic goes:

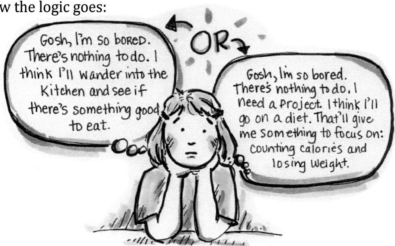

The Solution

There are lots of smart actions that help with boredom that do not involve *eating or not eating*. Here are a few ideas:

Draw a picture, write a letter to a friend, do a puzzle, rearrange the shoes in your closet, crank up some music and dance, sing a song, write in a journal, read a book, play with your dog, dress up your cat.

your turn

OK, now it's your turn. Come up with ten things that do not involve a screen that you can do when you are bored besides EAT or NOT EAT.

1.

2.

3.

4.

5.

6.

7.

8.

9.

10.

Awesome Quotes About Boredom

Boredom is the feeling that everything is a waste of time; serenity, that nothing is.

–Thomas Szasz

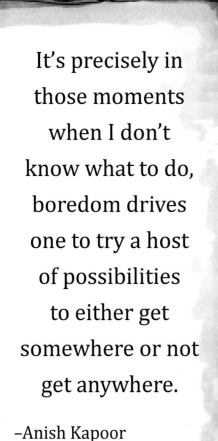

It's precisely in those moments when I don't know what to do, boredom drives one to try a host of possibilities to either get somewhere or not get anywhere.

–Anish Kapoor

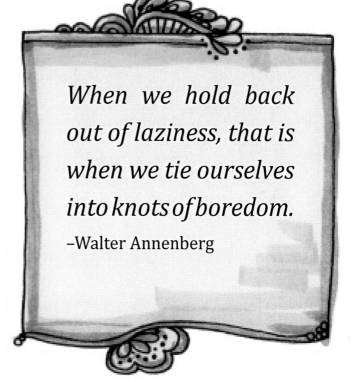

When we hold back out of laziness, that is when we tie ourselves into knots of boredom.

–Walter Annenberg

You'll find boredom where there is the absence of a good idea.

–Earl Nightingale

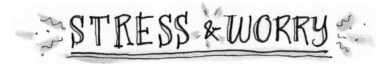
STRESS & WORRY

The Problem

These days there are plenty of problems, big and small, that are creating stress in our lives. The bad economy has been tough on many families, and there is nothing that stresses a kid like stressed parents! Even if your parents don't have money stress, there is plenty of stress in a typical tween life: your friend loves you one day and disses you the next, there's that English test coming up, you're trying out for cheerleading, you have to memorize your lines for the school play by tomorrow. Mean kids, cyber-bullying, annoying siblings, arguing parents—the list of things that cause stress is long. Plus, add to that the changes in your body due to hormones. Did you know that hormonal changes make you feel more emotional? (In other words, tweens tend to feel angrier, sadder and more upset than normal because of these hormones. Thanks a lot, Hormones!)

BUT— here's an interesting fact about stress:

You can change your stress level by changing your thoughts. Are you a worrier? Do you take a situation and imagine the worst possible scenario that could happen and then convince yourself that it's definitely going to happen?

Example: I didn't have enough time to study for this test. I am going to fail this test. My teachers and my parents will be mad at me. My grade point average will drop. I will not get into the college of my choice. I will not be successful or happy in life. HELP!

Example: My friend seemed kind of cold to me today. Maybe she hates me. Maybe she is going to turn everyone against me. She is going to make up stories about me and everyone is going to hate me. I won't be able to tell any adults or I'll be called a tattle-tale. I will be forever alone and lonely. HELP!

99% of the time, the thing that you are stressed and worried about does not happen. You can see how worrying about the most awful possibility can cause you lots of stress! It is actually a relief to know that your own thoughts can increase or decrease your stress, because that means you can actually do something about it!

Stress and worry, like boredom, can be at the root of eating problems. Here's how it works:

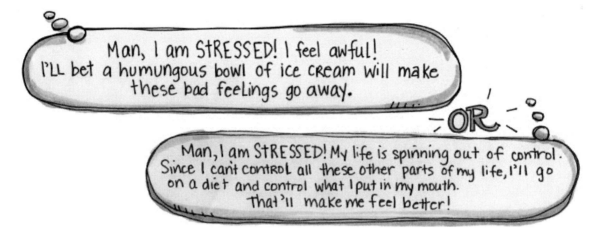

Eating or dieting may both make you feel better for a little while, but they may only be distractions that last for a few minutes. Even worse, they often cause you more problems than you had in the first place: weight problems, self-esteem problems, stomach aches, lack of energy, and lots of wasted time; more problems which only add to your stress.

The Solution

Remember we talked about finding the smartest action to match up the feeling with the need? There are lots of smart actions that help with stress that don't involve food. The smart actions that help with boredom are often great for stress, too. Here are a few ideas that help with stress:

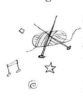

Lie on your bed and listen to music, stretch your muscles, dance, go for a jog, find someone to hug, knit, play cards, play an instrument. Talk about it. (Remember, sometimes stress is caused by thoughts in your head, so getting another viewpoint can help reassure you and calm you down.)

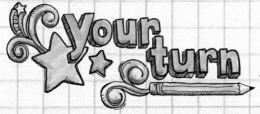

Come up with ten things that you can do when you are stressed besides EAT or NOT EAT.

1.

2.

3.

4.

5.

6.

7.

8.

9.

10.

Awesome Quotes about Stress & Worry

Worry does not empty tomorrow of its sorrow. It empties today of its strength.

–Corrie Ten Boom

While we are focusing on fear, worry, or hate, it is not possible for us to be experiencing happiness, enthusiasm or love.

–Bo Bennett

Most things I worry about never happen anyway.

–Tom Petty

My mother made it clear that you have to live life by your own terms and you have to not worry about what other people think and you have to have the courage to do the unexpected.

–Caroline Kennedy

My mother said, 'Don't worry about what people think now. Think about whether your children and grandchildren will think you've done well.'

–Lord Mountbatten

perfectionism

The Problem

Over the past twenty years, scientists have explored the mystery of who gets an eating disorder and who doesn't. They've put together some clues to solve this riddle. The one personality trait that tends to shows up in people who develop eating disorders is *perfectionism*.

It can be helpful to think of Perfectionism the same way we've been thinking about ED, like an annoying little voice inside of your head. A person who struggles with perfectionism is never happy for very long. She can't enjoy her accomplishments because Perfectionism says, "You could have done better." Perfectionism sets very high standards and tells you that you have to be the best. Perfectionism pushes you very hard!

You probably hear coaches, teachers, and parents say, "Do your best!" several times a day. On the one hand, setting a goal and working hard to achieve it is a formula for a successful life. Whether learning to pitch a strike in softball, playing a new piece of music on the piano, or mastering a new dance move, trying hard and doing your best will help you succeed!

On the other hand, be honest with yourself:

- Is your need to be the best getting out of hand?
- Are you losing sleep or getting stomach aches because you are so stressed?
- Have you become so obsessed with your goals (in grades or sports or appearance) that you can't hang out and relax without feeling guilty?
- When you do achieve your goal, does the good feeling disappear quickly because you feel pressure to maintain or even top your own accomplishment?

Take this quiz to see if you might be slipping into perfectionism.

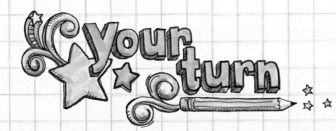

THE PERFECTIONISM QUIZ

Circle the first answer that comes to mind. We'll score it at the end.

1) The idea of being average is a terrible thought to me.

    a. I agree. I want to be above average.

    b. I don't really care one way or the other.

    c. I disagree. Being average is A-okay with me.

2) I believe that if I am perfect for my parents, they will never be upset with me.

    a. I agree. I try to be perfect to keep them happy.

    b. I don't really have an opinion about this one way or the other.

    c. I disagree. My parents do not need me to be perfect.

3) When I make a mistake, it bothers me for a long time.

    a. I agree. Sometimes it eats at me for hours or even days.

    b. No opinion on this one way or the other.

    c. I disagree. I'm pretty good at letting mistakes go.

4) I sometimes procrastinate on a school project because I'm so worried about needing to do it perfectly.

    a. I agree. Sometimes it's hard to even get started because I'm so stressed about it.

    b. No feeling one way or the other.

    c. I disagree. Doing projects doesn't stress me out; I just dive right in!

5) When I try something new for the first time, if I don't do well right away, I'm probably going to quit.

    a. I agree. I do not want to look stupid.

    b. No feeling one way or the other.

    c. I disagree. I kind of enjoy trying something new, even if I can't get it right the first time.

6) When I look at my appearance, I focus on the things I don't like about the way I look or things I'd like to change.

    a. I agree. I am not happy with what I see in the mirror.

    b. No feeling one way or the other.

    c. I disagree. I'm pretty happy with my appearance overall.

1) People say that I'm "hard to please."

    a. I agree. I hear this all the time.

    b. No feeling one way or the other .

    c. I disagree. In fact, I'm pretty easy to please,

2) When someone gives me constructive criticism, (in other words, tells me how I can do something better) it's very upsetting to me.

    a. I agree. It hurts my feelings to be criticized.

    b. No feeling one way or the other

    c. I disagree. I actually like hearing about how I can improve on something.

3) Sometimes no matter how well I do at something, I feel let down afterwards!

    a. I agree. It seems like I get my hopes up and then get disappointed.

    b. No feeling one way or the other.

    c. I disagree. I am generally okay with how things turn out.

4) When I look at something that I've done, I notice the little mistakes and little imperfections first.

    a. I agree. That's all I can notice.

    b. No feeling one way or the other.

    c. I disagree. I can see the overall good in the things that I do.

5) When I am focused on trying to achieve something, I keep my eye on the prize, always focusing on the final goal.

    a. I agree. Why bother doing something if you can't be the best?

    b. No feeling one way or the other.

    c. I disagree. I enjoy the process of doing things, even if I'm not the best.

6) If I get a 94 on a test, I'm going to be more focused on the 6 points I didn't get than on the 94 points I got right.

    a. I agree. It really upsets me when I don't get high A's.

    b. No feeling one way or the other.

    c. I disagree. I'd be pretty darn happy with a 94!

Results

SCORING: TOTAL

For every A, score = 2 points.   _____

For every B, score = 1 points   _____

For every C, score = 0 points   _____

(Let's add them up!)   TOTAL POINTS: _____

What does it mean?

0-15 points: *Non-Perfectionist*

You may set goals for yourself and be a high achiever, but you don't stress out about things too much. You are happy doing a good job, even if your goals aren't completely met. You take pride in your accomplishments and tend to be supportive of others. You enjoy the process of chasing a goal as much as reaching the goal itself. For example, if you are on the track team, you might enjoy running during practice and participating in meets, but you are okay if you don't win or reach a specific goal. You bounce back pretty quickly after a disappointment. You are cool with being coached, since you see it as helpful information that will improve your future performance.

16-24 points: *Perfectionist*

If you are a perfectionist, you tend to be too hard on yourself, focusing on tiny mistakes and imperfections. You believe if that you don't achieve your goals perfectly, then you've failed (even if you set goals that are too high!) Because you are so concerned about not failing, it's hard to enjoy the process of learning something, which involves making and learning from your mistakes. You believe that mistakes are not okay, and you may beat yourself up when you don't meet your high expectations. Sometimes you may avoid or put off working on a project because you are so afraid of it not being perfect. You also don't like constructive criticism because you are already so critical of yourself! Rather than enjoying your accomplishments, Perfectionism (like ED) comes along to ruin it ("You could have done better," or "You didn't really deserve that.")

The Solution

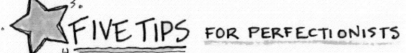

FIVE TIPS FOR PERFECTIONISTS

1. **Make an effort to focus on all the things that are good about whatever you do.** Instead of saying, "I only got a 94!" you can say, "Wow, A is for Awesome!"

2. **If you notice something you don't like about yourself, find five things that you do like.** Come on, you can find five things! Encourage yourself just like you would encourage a friend.

3. **Forgive yourself if you make mistakes.** Michael Jordan, the most awesome basketball player of all time, missed more than 9,000 shots in his career. He lost 300 games. Twenty-six times he was trusted to take the game-winning shot and missed.

4. **Set small, realistic goals for yourself.** You wouldn't yell at a baby for not knowing how to walk, would you? When you were a baby, you fell down a bunch of times before you started walking. What if you had given up because you didn't do it perfect the first time?

5. **Be open to constructive criticism.** See it as information that will help you improve. Just because you are not perfect, it doesn't mean you are awful! You are a "Work in Progress," just like the rest of us flawed humans.

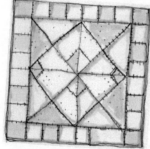

(Can you find the mistake?)

Amish quilters are known for the gorgeous, elegant quilts that they stitch by hand. But an Amish quilter always makes sure that one patch is WRONG! She adds one patch that is the wrong color or the wrong shape. "Why would someone mess up on purpose?" you might ask. The Amish believe that only God is perfect. Human beings are not supposed to be perfect. That Patch-Out-of-Place is to remind us to be humble about our imperfect selves.

And the most important thing to remember: If you are the child or sibling of someone with an eating disorder plus you are a perfectionist, *do not go on a diet.* The combination of your genetics and your perfectionism make it more likely that you could develop an eating disorder. Here's how Perfectionism turns a diet into an eating disorder. Start on a diet and Perfectionism will say, "You have to be the *best* dieter. You cannot mess up with your food. You have to do it perfectly! You have to be the skinniest girl in your class." Hmmmm...sound familiar? That's ED talking!

So, if you want to be healthy and happy, remember Michael Jordan missing those baskets and the Amish quilters putting in the wrong patch...and forget about perfectionism and dieting.

Awesome Quotes about Success & Failure

Perfectionism is not a quest for the best. It is a pursuit of the worst in ourselves, the part that tells us that nothing we do will ever be good enough.

–Julia Cameron

Success consists of going from failure to failure without loss of enthusiasm.

–Winston Churchill

I can accept failure, everyone fails at something. But I can't accept not trying.

–Michael Jordan

I honestly think it is better to be a failure at something you love than to be a success at something you hate.

–George Burns

All about Body Image

As we discussed earlier, body image only has a little bit to do with how your body actually looks. It's about how you see your body, and how you feel about what you see.

Sherry sees her body as a little bit larger than average. She's very happy and satisfied with the way she looks, because having a perfect body just doesn't matter that much to her.

Joey sees himself as a little bigger in some places and a little smaller in other places than he'd like to be, but it's really no big deal to him.

Sherry and Joey both have a positive body image.

Andrea thinks she is huge and disgusting and she is very sad about the fact that she thinks she's ugly. She is aware of her body size and thinks about it all day. She avoids beach trips, wears baggy clothes and puts herself down in front of her friends.

Bryan thinks he's too skinny. It seems most of his friends have started puberty and are developing muscles in their arms and chest. Bryan has started looking for pills that might help him get bigger and has started lifting weights to make himself more muscular.

If you met Andrea or Bryan, you'd think they look just fine. It can be hard to believe or understand why they are so unhappy with their bodies.

Body Image Influencers

Parents: The way your parents talk about bodies can affect you. Does your mom say that she feels fat? Does your dad make negative comments about the appearance of people on TV or in public?

Siblings: Comments by brothers and sisters can contribute to negative body image.

Mean kids: Did someone at school make a comment about your body, harass or bully you?

Friends: If you have a skinny friend, you may feel fat if you compare yourself to her. Do you have friends who spend a lot of time hating on their bodies or dieting?

The Media: If you watch lots of TV, play video games, spend time on Facebook, or look at magazines, you might compare your body to images and pictures that are not real or healthy.

Sports: Playing a sport can impact body image. While being fit and active can improve your body image, there are some sports that emphasize thinness and perfection (ballet, figure skating, gymnastics, cross-country running). These can actually harm body image.

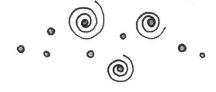

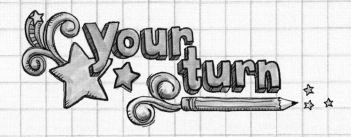

YOUR BODY IMAGE

Where are you on the body image chart?

1	2	3	4	5	6	7	8	9	10
Negative									**Positive**

Write about what you think has influenced your body image. Look at the list on the last page. Write about experiences that you've had, comments by others (positive or negative) about your body, comments that you've heard about other peoples' bodies, and any other things you believe have helped to create your body image.

If you have a positive body image, that's fantastic! Keep doing whatever you've been doing! But if your body image could be improved, write about some things that you appreciate about your body.

Body Image & Eating Disorders

If you have a positive body image, you will want to take care of your body! Taking care of your body means eating well, getting enough sleep and being physically active. All of these things help you feel good and help you look good.

But if you have a negative body image, you are more likely to do anything (even something harmful) to try to change your body so you'll think it looks better: things like starving yourself or making yourself vomit after you've eaten (you can see how an eating disorder can get started here). Your body will not be happy if you do these things!

When you HATE something you are not going to take very good care of it. Here are some Tips for Loving Your Body:

Do not compare yourself to others when it comes to body size and shape. As Lady Gaga says proudly, "I was born this way!" We are all supposed to look and be different ... and that's a good thing!

Don't spend a lot of time looking at pictures in magazines or comparing yourself to models and actresses. The images you see have been created on a computer and they are not what the person really looks like. Many super-thin actresses are miserable and struggling with eating disorders.

Appreciate your body for what it does instead of how it looks. Don't you feel great when you go for a run or play a sport? Doesn't it feel good to dance or go hiking in the woods? Think about people who are ill or disabled and would love to have a body that is capable of doing all that your body does for you. A sense of appreciation is an important part of feeling good about yourself!

You-Pie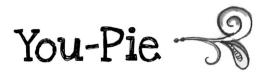

Think of yourself as a pie. There are many delicious slices in this You-Pie. Each slice represents an important part of who you are.

Here is an example of some of the slices of a you-pie!

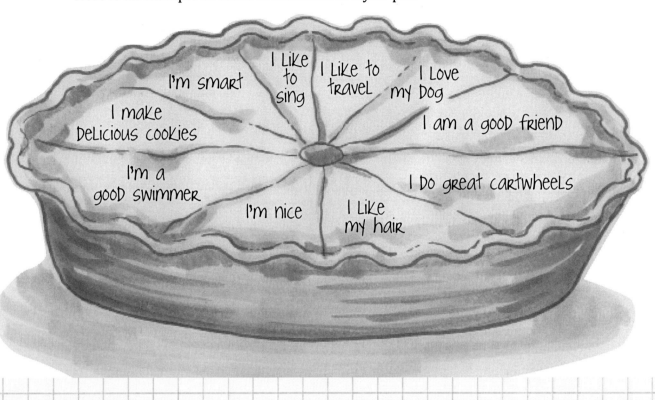

Fill in the pie below with some of the things that describe you.

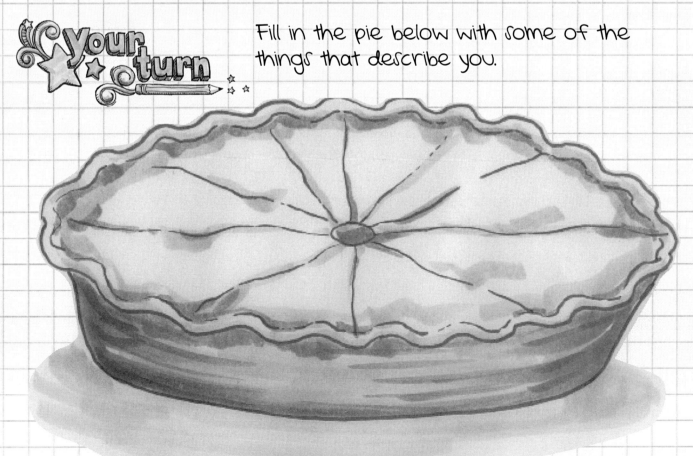

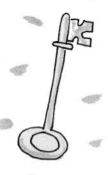

When you think about who you are, it's important to realize that the way you look is just one slice of the You-Pie!

If appearance takes up too many slices, then you are missing out on the most delicious and wonderful parts of the pie! I can guarantee that the people who know and love you would not say that your appearance is the most interesting or special thing about you! But let's say that you think your appearance is the most interesting and special thing about you (in other words, it's taking up lots of slices of You-Pie). One morning you wake up feeling unhappy about how you look: your hair is lumpy in the back, your socks don't match, your clothes are too tight, or you have a pimple on your chin (and, believe me, we all have those days). If your appearance takes up a bunch of slices of the You-Pie then you are going to have one lousy rotten day. But if your appearance only takes up just one little slice, then you'll think, "Oh, well. Nobody's perfect! I'm still pretty awesome!" and you'll face your day with a positive attitude! Just one good reason for just one slice.

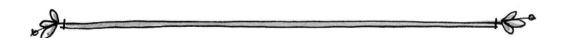

Awesome Quotes about Body & Beauty

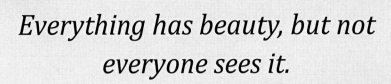

Everything has beauty, but not everyone sees it.

–Confucius

Since love grows within you, so beauty grows. For love is the beauty of the soul.

–Saint Augustine

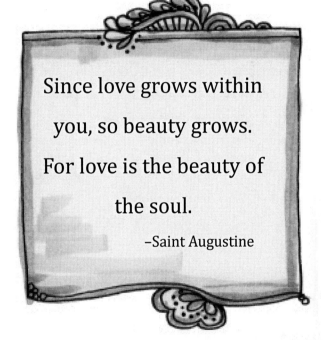

Inner beauty should be the most important part of improving one's self.

–Priscilla Presley

Beauty is how you feel inside, and it reflects in your eyes. It is not something physical.

–Sophia Loren

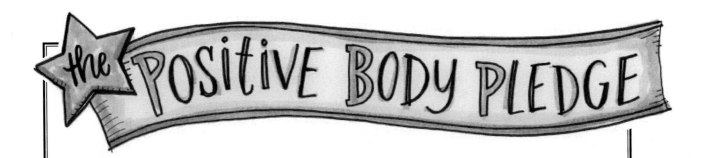

the POSITIVE BODY PLEDGE

- I will say kind things to and about my body.

- I will not use eating or not eating to make bad feelings go away.

- I will move my body so I can be fit, healthy, strong and happy.

- I will do my best, knowing it's okay to not be perfect.

- I will deal with worrying by talking to others, getting reassurance, finding comfort and trying to relax.

- I will find creative and positive ways to deal with stress and boredom.

- I will not engage in Fat Talk ("I'm so fat!" "She's so fat!") with my friends.

- I will think of things that I appreciate about my body.

- I will not diet, especially if I'm related to a person with an eating disorder.

- If I hear the voice of ED in my head or in the head of my friends, I will speak to an adult and get help.

Name

Date

_____   _____

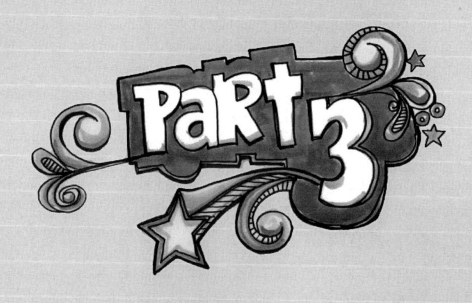

When Someone You Love Has an Eating Disorder

So...

Now you know. A person you love has an eating disorder. Maybe you figured it out by watching her. Like a detective, you put together the clues.

- She's been looking a lot thinner these days.

- She eats lots of salads and won't eat what everyone else is having.

- She avoids dessert at parties.

- She has to go for a run every day or she's in a terrible mood.

- Or maybe you noticed that she's gained weight lately.

- You discovered her secretly eating ice cream after saying she wasn't going to have any.

- Or you heard her throwing up in the bathroom.

Perhaps your friend told you that she's been throwing up lunch and begged you to keep her secret. Perhaps your parents sat you down and explained that your mother or your sister has an eating disorder. Now you have this new big piece of information. Your heart is pounding and your stomach is fluttering. Your head is spinning with questions you can't even put into words.

Part Three will answer lots of your questions about how to cope with this situation. The most important thing for you to know is that you are not alone. Because there are millions of people with eating disorders, that means there are millions of tweens just like you, feeling the same feelings and asking the same questions. The information in Part Three will help you to help yourself and the person you love.

How You Can Help

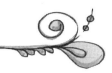

The first thing you need to understand is that *this is not your fault.* Humans love to simplify things, but eating disorders are extremely complicated. We wish we could point to one thing and say, "*That* caused my loved one to get an eating disorder!" If that were true, it might be a whole lot easier to fix. But the cause of an eating disorder is different for every person. It's a result of a mysterious combination of the DNA that she inherited, personality traits, family stress, peer influences, food restriction, and unhealthy messages in the media. The truth is that there is nothing that you ever did or said that caused her to have an eating disorder. In fact, no person in the history of the world has ever given another person an eating disorder.

So please don't waste one minute of your precious time blaming yourself. Thank you.

The Sad Truth

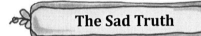

As much as you wish you could make it all better, you can't fix this problem.

- You wish you could say *the magic words* and she'd wake up tomorrow without an eating disorder.

- You wish you could give her *the perfect love-filled hug* and everything would feel better inside of her.

- You wish you could give her *the most delicious treat* and then the spell would be broken.

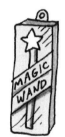

Unfortunately, most adults don't even know how to solve an eating disorder, so don't expect that you should be able to fix this. She will get better by working with adults who have special training and education in eating disorders.

The Happy Truth

So even though gifts of words and hugs and food cannot *fix* her problem, they really do *help.* (Well, words and hugs for now, maybe food a little later!) So keep offering these wonderful gifts! *Love* is one of the most important ingredients in recovery.

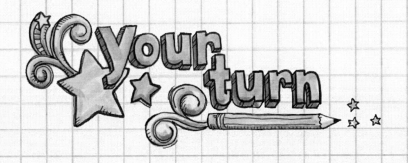

Get some paper, markers, or paint.
Write or draw words or pictures that
describe the way you see your loved
one: beautiful, kind, loving, funny, a great
hugger, whatever words come to you.

Write down the things they have done
or said that make them special to you.
Give these to her and she will read them
over and over to remind herself of how
you feel about her.

Seeing herself through the eyes of those
who love her will help your loved one
heal from her eating disorder.

Why Did She Get One?

A person with an eating disorder is usually super-smart and extra-sensitive. She has a strong sense of *right* and *wrong*. Because of this, she is very tuned in to situations that feel bad or sad, such as mean girls at school, arguments between her parents, the loss of a pet, or the stress of a sick relative. Because we live in an imperfect world, she tends to worry about the things that she sees around her. There are two ways she tries to cope with her imperfect world:

1. *She tries to fix the situation **outside** of her.*

2. *She tries to fix the bad feelings **inside** of her.*

To fix the *outside* situation, she works hard to make people happy. One way to please others is to be perfect! Whether keeping her room neat, getting good grades or excelling in sports, she tries to make others proud and happy. Perhaps she thought, "I'll feel better about myself if I lose a couple of pounds," or "I'll be healthier if I stop eating fried food and sweets." But when a perfectionist goes on a diet, she's never happy. The voice of ED says: "Sure, you lost some weight, but think how good you'll feel if you lose even more..." ED rarely lets her feel good about her body.

To fix the *inside* situation, she has to find a way to make her negative feelings go away. She may have been told that anger and sadness are "Not ladylike," "Not nice," or even "ugly." So instead of talking about her feelings, she'll smile and say, "I'm fine," even when she isn't. She may have discovered that overeating or restricting her food quiet the painful feelings. Eating or not eating give her a temporary lift and cause her bad feelings to go numb.

What do I mean by go numb?

Have you ever gone to the dentist to get a cavity filled? The dentist gave you a shot to numb your cheek so you didn't feel any pain. Being numb means you can't feel pain.

However, this method of eating or not eating to numb painful feelings is only a temporary solution. Eventually bad feelings return! The more she uses eating or not eating to cope, the farther away she gets from knowing who she is and what she feels. She stopped taking care of her body because she was more focused on numbing the painful emotions of sadness, anger and worry. Over time this way of coping turned into an eating disorder.

After weeks or months or years of ignoring her body and her feelings, it can be difficult to learn these things. However, the good news is that it's never too late! It may take time and professional help, but she can get better. It's also important to know that your loved one probably did not DECIDE to have an eating disorder. She didn't think, "Wow, I have these bad feelings inside. I think I'll restrict my food to see if that makes me feel better." It probably started as an innocent little diet that took on a life of its own.

Building Your Support Team

Finding out that someone you love has an eating disorder is a tough piece of information to digest. Even though much of the attention will be focused on your loved one, you'll have questions that need answering and feelings that you need to express, too! You may need to talk to someone if you're confused, scared, or angry or if you just need a hug! Check out this list, then put together your own list!

Your Mom, Dad, Step-Mom or Step-Dad   A therapist
Your Grandma, Your Aunt or Your cousin Your brother or sister
A Parent of a friend   Your best friend
Your school counselor   Other Kids with Loved ones with eating Disorders.
Your teacher

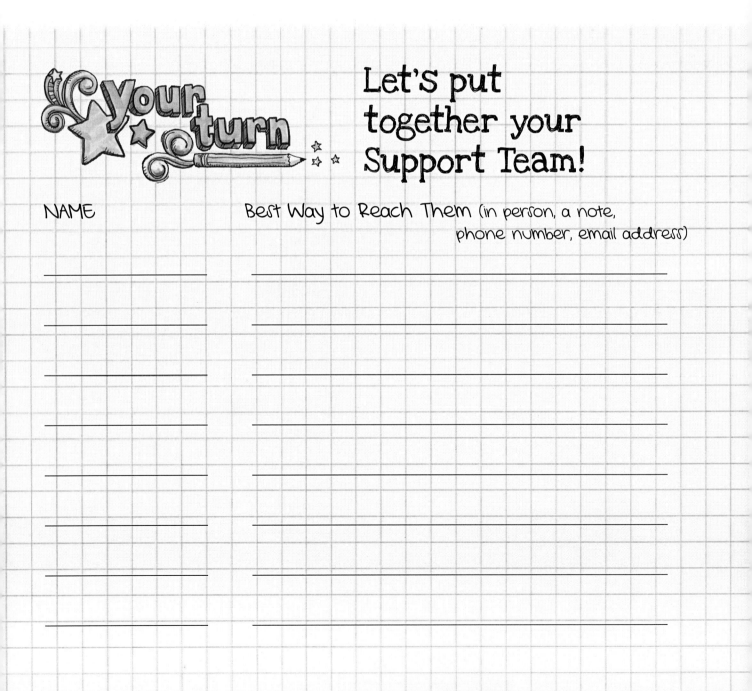

Let's put together your Support Team!

NAME   Best Way to Reach Them (in person, a note, phone number, email address)

_____   _____

_____   _____

_____   _____

_____   _____

_____   _____

_____   _____

_____   _____

What You Might Be Feeling

If someone you love is struggling with an eating disorder, you are probably having a tough time, too! These are some of the very normal and completely understandable emotions that you may be feeling.

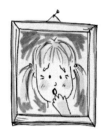

Scared & Worried: It can be scary to see someone you love dealing with an eating disorder and feel like there's nothing you can do to stop it. Her body may have changed. Her personality may have changed. It's like an evil force has brainwashed her, taken possession of her body and is hurting her from the inside (Exactly! His name is ED).

If she's your friend or your younger sister, you may worry that you can't protect her. What if someone at school says something stupid or she sees something on TV that causes her ED to get worse?

If she's the older sister whom you seek out when you're having a bad day, you may feel worried that she's not there to look out for you.

It can be especially scary if your mom has an eating disorder. We see our parents as strong and capable. It's tough to realize that your mom isn't perfect, and that she is dealing with emotional struggles. You may be especially worried about who's going to take care of you if she needs to go to a treatment center.

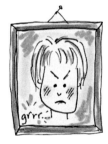

Angry: You may find yourself feeling angry. Angry that she won't eat. Angry that she's eating too much. Angry that she's causing so much turmoil in your social life or in your home. "How can she do this? Doesn't she care about what this is doing to me?"

You may feel angry at ED for stealing your friend or your sister or your mother, especially if she has to go away to a treatment center.

You may look for someone or something to blame: if you could figure out whose "fault" it is, then you'd have a place to focus your anger. If your mom is sick, you may blame your dad: "How could he let this happen to her?"

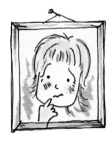

Confused: It's normal to wonder, "How did this happen?" Eating disorders are so complicated and don't make sense. You may wonder, "How can she just suddenly stop eating?" or "Why does she think she's fat when she's not?" If your loved one is a family member, it's confusing to see everyone in your home under such stress. It's like ED snuck up and dropped a bomb in the middle of your kitchen table.

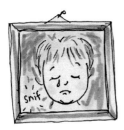

Sad: Whenever something big changes in a person's life, it is normal to feel sad. You miss the way things used to be. You may even burst into tears sometimes. These waves of sadness can sneak up when you least expect it. If your loved one has to go to a treatment center, you may feel sad that she'll miss your sports events or performances. If it's your mom, you'll miss her tucking you into bed and giving you hugs.

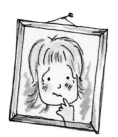

Guilty: Kids your age often take things personally, even when it's not their fault. You may feel guilty, wondering if there was something you did or didn't do that caused this. "Maybe if I had gotten better grades, she would have been happy and this wouldn't have happened!" "Maybe if I had been a better friend, she wouldn't have gotten bulimia." You may even feel guilty for feeling angry: "How can I be mad at her when it's not her fault? I must be a terrible person!"

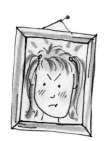

Envy: You probably think your friend or loved one is beautiful. You may even think, "Hmmm, maybe if I got an eating disorder, I'd be as beautiful as she is!" You may feel envious that she is getting lots of attention (even if it's negative attention). You may even think, "Hmmm, maybe if I stopped eating or started throwing up, someone would pay attention to me around here..." (Hopefully reading this book will help with the feelings of envy. It should become crystal clear that an eating disorder only brings misery and unhappiness and that it's the last thing on earth that you would want!)

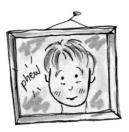

Relief: Finding out your loved one has an eating disorder may actually be a relief! It helps explain things you noticed but didn't understand. Suddenly it all makes sense. It's nice to know you weren't crazy when you noticed things weren't right: mystery solved! Also, if you know that she's getting help, then you can breathe easier. If she goes to an inpatient treatment center, you can send her emails and letters, talk to her on the phone or even visit her. If things have been tense with her around, you may feel relieved that she is going away. Feeling this way does not mean that you are a bad person; it just means that it's very hard to be around ED!

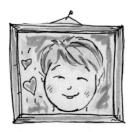

Pure Love: You may feel very powerful feelings of love for your friend, sister, or mom as she is going through all this. The entire experience might actually get everyone talking more openly and make everyone feel closer and more connected! You may be able to sense the helplessness and pain that your loved one is experiencing and feel a strong compassion for her.

Best Ways to Deal With These Feelings

It's important for you to be able to express the feelings that you have inside. If your loved one is a family member, you may be able to talk to your parents about these feelings since they are closest to the situation and they are the most likely people to understand exactly what you're going through.

On the other hand, sometimes parents are so stressed out that you might not get the response you need from them.

They may say something like: "That's ridiculous! Stop feeling that way!" or "I can't believe you are being so selfish at a time like this. This is not about you!" While they may be making these comments to try to stop you from feeling bad, it doesn't really work, does it? It may just make you feel another bad feeling on top of your first bad feeling! ("Great, so now I'm angry and selfish!")

If you think your parents might react negatively to your feelings, find an adult on your support team to contact. You noticed I said *adult.* While talking to your friends can be helpful, these situations are extremely complicated and you need an adult's perspective.

Sometimes putting your thoughts and feelings on paper helps you feel better and see things in a new light. The next *Your Turn* section is a place to write about what you're experiencing. If there's not enough space, use a private journal or notebook. After that, there is a place for you to draw your own picture of ED!

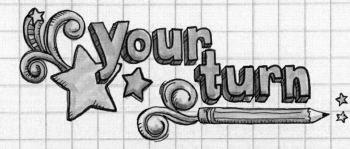

Write about the feelings that you are having. You can start here, but if there's more to write, get a journal where you can write more about your feelings.

My feelings:

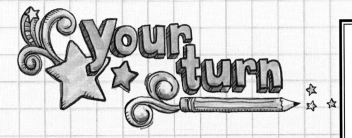

ASK YOUR LOVED one if she has a name for her eating DISORDER. If not, the two of you can come UP with one.

(WRITE it here)

It's helpful to be able to refer to the eating DISORDER Like this because it reminds you (and her) that she is not her eating DISORDER

You can say things Like, "HEY, ED, stop bullying my mom/sister! she's awesome! I'm sick of you making her feel bad! I Love her!"

Draw a picture of what you think ED looks like:

More Healthy Ways to Express and Soothe Feelings

Remember in the section about ED, I explained that an eating disorder is a way to numb uncomfortable feelings.

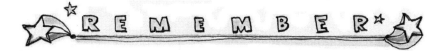

> **Eating** or **not eating** are dangerous coping mechanisms. The best way to try to prevent yourself from getting an eating disorder is to find healthy ways to express feelings.

We have already mentioned two ways: talking with someone and writing it down. There are other great ways to express painful feelings: poetry, art, and dance are just a few.

It's also okay to distract yourself from bad feelings by doing something to get your mind off of them: play with your dog, watch a hilarious comedy, hang out with your friends. You don't want to get stuck in your bad feelings all day long. It's okay to just take a break. (Remember on page 41 you came up with healthy ways to deal with stress and worry.)

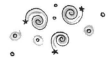

Taking Action

What Not To Do

If you suspect that a person you love has an eating disorder, but she won't admit it...

1. Don't go on a diet with her as this will only make her unhealthy behavior seem OK to her. After all, you're doing it together!

2. Don't Binge or Purge with her (for the same reason). Sometimes people with eating disorders invite their friends to join them so their behavior seems more normal.

3. Don't promise to keep her secret if her eating problems make you uncomfortable. As you've discovered, these problems can be dangerous and hard to fix. You may need to tell an adult so she can get help. Telling an adult doesn't make you a "Tattle-Tale." It makes you a "Loving Friend" and possibly even a "Life-Saver."

What To Do

1. If she has not told anyone yet, offer to go with her to talk to your parents, the school counselor, or another trusted adult. She may be more willing to go if you offer to go with her.

2. Find things to do together that have nothing to do with food or body size. Paint each other's toe-nails, go see a funny movie together, play board games or take a walk. These activities can give her a break from the bad feelings and give you both a break from ED. As she starts her recovery, she'll need positive memories and messages to fight ED. The best gift you can give her is the knowledge that she is loved and that she matters.

3. If the stress of the relationship is too much for you, then it's okay to take a break from it. If being around her makes you feel anxious, depressed or helpless, you may need some time away from her. You can't be helpful if you're miserable!

What Not to Say

1. Try not to say, "Your stupid eating disorder is really making me angry!" ED will say to her, "See, you're a terrible person. Look how much pain you're causing everyone!"

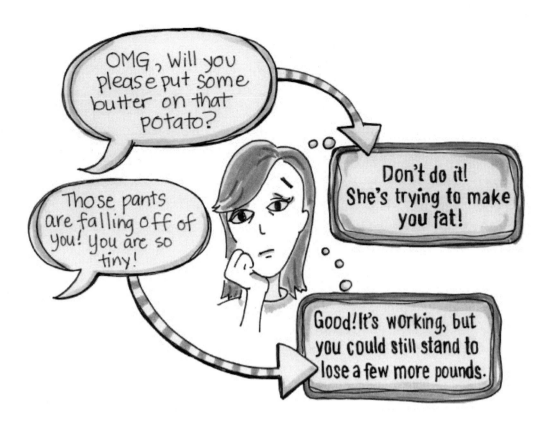

2. If you say, "You're getting sooo skinny and it's really scaring me!" ED will hear "sooo skinny" and think, "Yay, it's working! Great job!" (She won't be able to hear the "it's really scaring me" part.) If she starts to recover and her weight changes, don't say, "You look so much healthier! " ED will hear, "You are HUGE!"

3. Try not to talk about the food she's eating. "Wow, your dietician lets you eat all that? You're so lucky!" ED will hear, "You are a gross, out-of-control PIG!" Remember, even though an eating disorder seems like it's about food and weight, it's really about poor self-esteem and coping with negative feelings.

What To Say:

You may be wondering whether you should share your feelings with your loved one. Well, it depends!

When a person is just starting their recovery, it may be hard for her to hear how you feel. ED makes everything about her: anything negative from the outside will be used to beat her up.

But as she starts to recover, she may be better at hearing feedback from others.

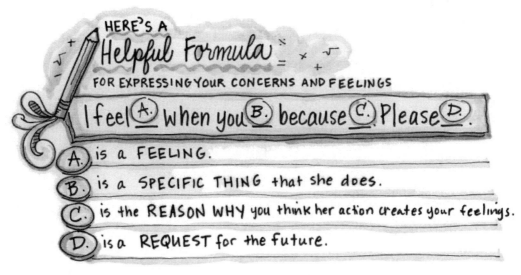

HERE'S A **Helpful Formula** FOR EXPRESSING YOUR CONCERNS AND FEELINGS

I feel (A.) when you (B.) because (C.) Please (D.).

(A.) is a FEELING.

(B.) is a SPECIFIC THING that she does.

(C.) is the REASON WHY you think her action creates your feelings.

(D.) is a REQUEST for the future.

For example:

I feel scared **when you** throw up after lunch **because** I care about you and I'm worried about your health. **Please** try not to throw up lunch when we eat together.

I feel sad **when you** pick fights with Dad about food at the dinner table **because** you need to eat dinner in order to get better. **Please** try not to fight at dinner.

This way of expressing yourself is called "Assertiveness." It is respectful of your feelings and it is respectful of the other person. She may not like to hear what you're saying, and she may not make the changes that you request, but at least she will start to see how people she loves are affected by her actions. Eventually there will come a day when realizing that her actions impact others will mean, "Hey, I matter! I need to take care of myself because people love me."

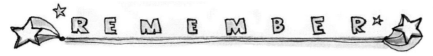

R E M E M B E R

Even though it may appear that she cannot hear your love, deep inside she is listening.

Even though an eating disorder seems like it's about food and weight, it's really about poor self-esteem and coping with negative feelings.

The best way to get your feelings out and help your loved one at the same time is to share your loving and concerned feelings with her. Even though it may appear that she cannot hear your love, deep inside she is listening. When you catch her in a sweet moment, say, "You are so funny and smart. I love you!"

How She'll Get Better

Because an eating disorder involves the body, spirit, and mind, there may be several different parts to her recovery process.

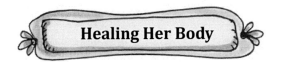 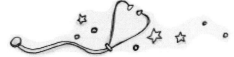

Healing Her Body

Medical Doctor Your loved one might work with a doctor who prescribes medication which helps soothe and calm the worrying and sadness that she feels inside. She also may be checked by a doctor who will make sure that her body is healthy. She may take vitamins to give her body an extra boost of nutrition.

Nutrition Counseling Because the eating disorder makes it hard for your loved one to know what, when and how much to eat, she may work with a Dietician or a Nutritionist. This person knows everything there is to know about food and the human body. The dietician will help her come up with a healthy eating plan full of nutritious and delicious food that will help her mind and body feel better and work better.

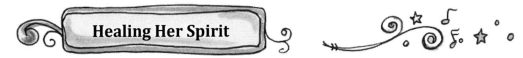

Healing Her Spirit

Art, Music & Movement Because she has used her eating disorder to make bad feelings go away, recovery will involve learning new ways to recognize and express her feelings. Art, music, and movement are great ways to do this! Part of her therapy may involve working with different forms of art such as painting, drawing, sculpture, or collage. She may find that listening to or creating music helps her get in touch with her feelings. She may be practicing new ways to move her body that are gentle and kind, such as yoga, meditation, or different types of dance. While it can be a little scary to try something new, these experiences will help her get to know herself better and become more confident in herself!

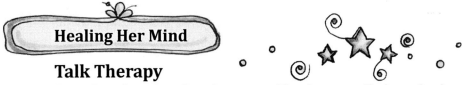

Healing Her Mind

Talk Therapy

Even though eating disorders seem like they are all about food and weight, they are also about thoughts and feelings. She can talk to a person such as a therapist, psychologist or counselor who will help her sort out the thoughts and feelings that are part of her eating disorder. The therapist might also invite other family members to the therapy sessions since everyone is affected by the eating disorder.

In therapy, your loved one will work on solving the mystery of why she developed this eating disorder. She will discover the ways that her eating disorder has helped her to cope with her problems in the past. Then she will be learning new healthier ways to cope with her feelings, *without* doing the things that ED tells her to do (such as *eat or not eat*).

As she gets better, she'll start sticking up for herself more in her relationships with others. She'll also be sticking up for herself inside of her own head:

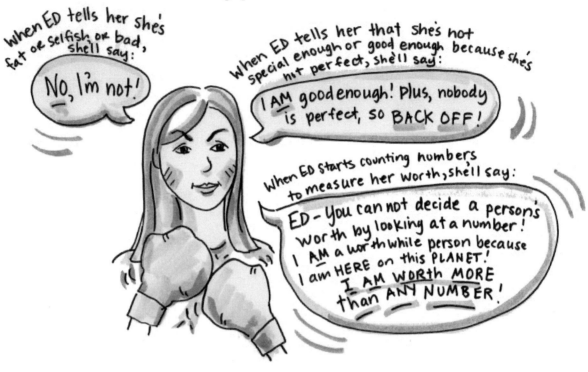

If She Needs to Go Away

If her eating disorder is seriously harming her health, she may need to go to an inpatient treatment facility for a few weeks or months. Inpatient treatment means that she is a patient who sleeps in the treatment center. Going away will be hard and scary. She'll miss the people she loves, but it will give her the chance to focus her attention on getting better. An inpatient treatment center is like a hospital with doctors, nurses and therapists, but it may look like a hotel or even a cozy home.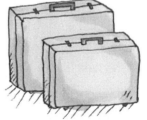

(You can probably see pictures on the treatment center's website.) She'll be eating great food because treatment centers hire excellent chefs who cook healthy delicious meals! She'll get to know other people with eating disorders and work with them in therapy groups. They'll help each other by giving advice, support and plenty of love. Because she's felt such shame about her problem, she hasn't shared her secret with many people. Finally it'll feel safe to talk openly about something that she's held inside for a long time. It will also be healing for her to grow closer to others who have this same problem. She'll feel like she's not the only one. That helps a lot!

A Special Case: When It's Mom

It can be very upsetting to find out that your mother has an eating disorder. She is the most important woman in your life and you love her very much. Hopefully the fact that you are reading this book means that she is getting help from professionals. Sometimes, families don't talk to the kids about a parent's eating disorder until it's gotten so serious that she has to get treatment. If she's suffering enough that she needs to go to inpatient treatment, then you get hit with *two* pieces of bad information at the same time:

1. Your mom is not okay, and
2. Your mom is going away to a treatment center for a while.

Message from a guy whose mom struggled with an eating disorder

MESSAGE

TO: *You*
From: *Tom*

I'm grown up now, but when I was a kid and for years after I grew up, my mom had an eating disorder. It was never talked about because we were frightened about confronting her. The pain and suffering she endured mentally and physically took its toll on her and the entire family. The secrecy, shame and guilt were overwhelming. I didn't know where to turn for help. This book is wonderful! I wish when I was a kid there had been a guide like this to help me and my family fully understand what was happening with our mom. She loved us so much, but her bulimia, over-exercising and constant purging destroyed her. An eating disorder is like that pink elephant in the room that everyone sees but pretends is not there. I hope this book will allow you to keep talking openly about your feelings and that your body is filled with love, light and healing.

Love, Tom

Making Plans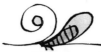

If your mom is going away, make a list of some of the things that Mom does for you. Then come up with ideas for what's going to happen while she's away. If there are items that you're unsure about, discuss these with your parents. You may think of things that they haven't even considered! (I filled in the first one for you.)

What Mom Does	While She's Away
Makes my breakfast	Dad can do it (pancakes) or I can do it (cereal)

What to Tell Others

Your friends may have noticed changes in your Mom's weight or appearance. They may want to know why she is going away. Ask your parents how they'd like you to handle these types of questions from your friends. Some families are very open and they will feel comfortable with you sharing this information with people in your life. Your teacher may encourage you to share your story with the class so they will learn more about eating disorders and be supportive to you. It can be comforting to know there are people who know the whole story so you can reach out to them if you're struggling with difficult thoughts or feelings. However, sometimes adults feel embarrassed or ashamed about a family member with an eating disorder or they may decide that this is a private family matter. If this is the case, ask your parents how they'd like you to handle questions from friends or teachers.

Unfortunately, many people do not understand eating disorders. Some people think that an eating disorder is the sufferer's fault. Others may view an eating disorder as a weakness or a choice instead of an illness. The best way to teach people about eating disorders is to educate them. Thankfully people are becoming more open about this topic.

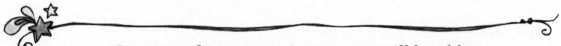

Because of your experiences, you will be able to raise awareness and increase understanding of eating disorders for the rest of your life.

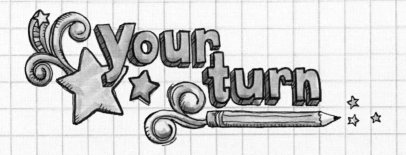

Once you've discussed this with your parents, write below who you can talk to and how you'll answer questions about your Mom's appearance, weight, and treatment:

Person   What I will say:

_____   _____

_____   _____

_____   _____

_____   _____

_____   _____

_____   _____

_____   _____

_____   _____

_____   _____

_____   _____

_____   _____

Message from a mom who struggles with an eating disorder

MESSAGE

To: You
From: Kara

Having an eating disorder is very scary for the whole family. I can see now, looking back, that it was overwhelming for my kids to see me in such an unhealthy state. At the time, I knew I wanted to get better for my three beautiful children, but my Eating Disorder was so powerful that I could not win this battle on my own. My children would express their concern to me and ask me questions about why I was so thin or why I didn't want to eat. I never knew how to answer them. Recovering from an eating disorder is a long, hard struggle. It is my hope that this book will provide some answers and support for you. As you read this book, it is my hope that you will remember how much your loved one cares for you and loves you and wants recovery so she can be the best parent or sibling for you.

~Kara

What About Dad?

Your Dad will probably have mixed feelings about your mom going to treatment, too. On the one hand, he'll feel relieved that she's getting help for her eating disorder. If he's been feeling tension and stress during meal times, he may breathe a sigh of relief that ED will no longer be joining the family for dinner.

However, he'll probably be nervous about juggling all the parent jobs while she is away. He may ask family members or friends to help get the kids to school and other activities. You might notice that he seems more stressed since his family-work *doubles* when she's away. The best way to support your dad during this time is to pick up after yourself and help out around the house. If you have younger brothers or sisters, try hard to get along and support each other. Depending on what's needed, you may want to learn how to start the washing machine, how to fill the dishwasher and even how to prepare simple meals. Whether these are new skills for you or whether you've been doing these things for years, it will feel good to help out in this way. Every member of the family can support in your mother's recovery by helping out around the house. And remember if you are having a tough time, Dad is on your support team. Go find him if you need some love and reassurance.

Every member of the family can assist in your mother's recovery by helping out with running the household.

During your mother's recovery, her relationship with your dad may change. Sometimes when a woman has an eating disorder, she and her husband argue a lot *before* she goes to treatment. It's almost like your dad is arguing with ED,

Go away! I want my wife back!

After treatment, with ED less involved in their lives, they may get along a lot better.

On the other hand, sometimes ED keeps a woman quiet in her marriage. ED says to her, "You are not worthy. Your needs don't matter." After treatment, she may start speaking up for herself more.

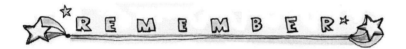

While this may be a good thing, it may mean that your parents argue more after she gets back from treatment.

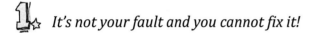

Often married couples who are having a hard time with this transition will work with a therapist to help them learn better ways to communicate and feel closer.

I know that hearing your parents argue can be very stressful!

☆ R E M E M B E R ☆

1. *It's not your fault and you cannot fix it!*

2. *It's normal for marriages to go through a tough time when one person has an eating disorder.*

3. *It will take some time for your parents to create a marriage without ED.*

4. *Remember to reach out to your support team if their problems are adding too much stress to your life. You are not alone!*

When She Gets Home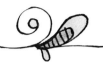

It's impossible to predict exactly how your loved one might be different after inpatient treatment. Every experience is unique, but these are some changes you might notice.

- She'll be super happy to see you again. She missed you and will be giving you lots of hugs when she returns!

- She'll look healthier than when she left. They've taken very good care of her, making sure she gets rest, great food, physical activity, and lots of love.

- Even though she'll feel stronger and more energetic, she may have trouble adjusting to her body if her weight has changed. She may still hear ED telling her she's fat (although the voice of ED might not be quite as loud as before).

- She may be eating and exercising differently when she returns home. She may eat foods that you haven't seen her eat before! She may be exercising more or less, depending upon which is healthier. This may still be difficult, but she'll be trying to hold onto the progress she made while she was away.

- She'll have healthier ways of coping with her feelings. She may seem calmer and more confident. You may find that she speaks up for herself and expresses her opinions more.

- She may still struggle with ED when she returns, perhaps for months or even years! Going away can help her learn to eat more normally. It can help her body become healthier and teach her helpful skills for coping with her feelings. However, she'll need to continue treatment even when she returns. She may slip back into some of her old habits at times. Don't be alarmed, but do share your concerns if you are worried about what you see.

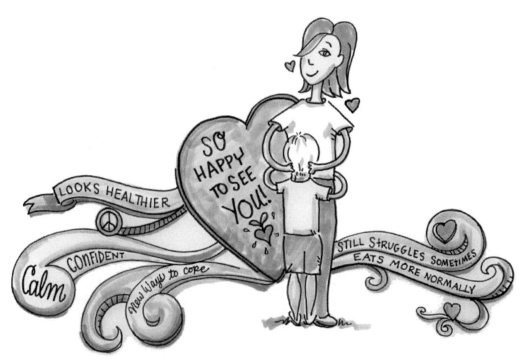

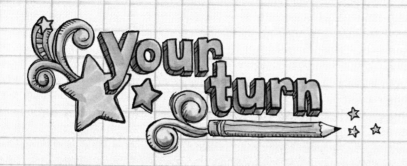

You can add to this list by writing down other ways that your loved one has changed since starting treatment for her eating disorder:

Real Questions from Tweens

Because this is such a complicated topic, in this section I'm going to answer some questions that kids have asked me over the years.

Is an eating disorder contagious? ~Molly P. (age 11)

No, you cannot pick up an eating disorder from someone else, like picking up a cold or other virus. However, you can definitely be influenced by the eating habits of those around you. It's important, no matter where you are or who's sitting next to you, that you stay focused on the signals in your own stomach. Everyone has a different body with different needs and appetites. Do not decide what you'll eat based on what other people are eating!

I'm a picky eater. Am I going to get an eating disorder? ~Cory L. (age 10)

Not necessarily. Lots of kids are picky. It's normal when you're young to be very sensitive to certain textures or flavors. Most kids grow out of pickiness as their taste buds mature and they start trying new foods. But some people remain picky eaters their whole lives.

On the other hand, some people are picky because they think certain foods are "bad." If a voice in your head is telling you that you aren't allowed to eat certain foods because they are bad (e.g. they have fat or carbohydrates in them or something else you think is scary) then you might want to talk to an adult. They can help you figure out if your picky eating may actually be the early sign of an eating disorder. If so, get some help turning it around as soon as possible!

I don't like eating in front of people. It just makes me uncomfortable. I feel like people are watching me eat. Is that normal? ~ Catherine P. (age 13)

Are you worried that other people think you're eating too much or not eating enough? Did someone say something to you about your eating? Or it may be that you worry too much about what others think, and you need to try to let go of those thoughts. Most people don't notice or care about what you eat! The most important thing to remember is to listen to the signals in your own body, and to ignore the comments that people make about your eating.

I love sweets and sometimes I sneak them into my room because my mom won't let me eat them? Is this a problem? ~Sarah C (age 11)

Why you are sneaking sweets? Are you hungry? That means you may not be eating enough at meals. Are you feeling something else? Lonely, sad or angry? Please read the section on Page 28about matching up food and feelings. You may be trying to comfort feelings other than hunger with food! You can learn better ways of matching up your feeling with what you really need. Are you sneaking sweets just because your parents have told you that you can't have them? Some families are so focused on being healthy that they don't allow sweets or treats in the house (especially when a mom has an eating disorder.) Talk to your parents about whether maybe you should be allowed to have dessert or a treat so you don't feel like you have to sneak it!

Sometimes I think it might be kind of nice to get an eating disorder. I think I might like the attention, people will be nicer to me, maybe I'll feel good about myself. I'm not so sure it's such a bad idea? ~ Jackie (age 10)

An eating disorder will affect every aspect of your life in a negative way. You will get attention, but it's not the kind of attention you'll enjoy. It's not fun to have people worried about you, upset with you or always watching you eat. There are many ways to get positive attention in life: doing good things, trying hard in school, being helpful to others. If living your life is like walking down a beautiful path, an eating disorder is like wandering off and getting lost in a dark and frightening forest.

It can be very lonely and scary and hard to find your way back to your life path. If you continue to have these thoughts and feelings, be sure to talk to your parents about it, and they will help you turn this around.

I'm bigger than all of my friends and I want to lose weight, but you're saying that dieting is bad. What am I supposed to do? ~ Isabel F. (age 12)

First, think about why you want to lose weight. Are you comparing yourself to your friends? Did someone make a comment about your body size? Losing weight is not the solution to either of these situations. Although it's hard, try to ignore the bodies and comments of people around you!

Second, you are at an age where people's bodies are changing fast. Many kids gain weight right before they have a growth spurt! Ask your parents if they gained weight right before they grew taller when they were your age. If that's what's happening, then please don't worry! You might be about to grow a few inches, and your body will naturally get thinner in the process.

But let's say that you have not been eating as healthy as you could, and maybe you are carrying extra weight because of it. First, I want you to think about these questions (also, see the section on Normal Eating on Page 20.) Do you keep eating even when you are full? Try to get better at listening to your belly when it says you are full. Do you eat when you are bored, stressed, lonely or sad? Read the section on Food & Feelings so you get better at taking care of those feelings in ways other than eating! Do you skip breakfast or lunch, and then eat most of your food when you get home from school until you go to bed? If you eat more at breakfast and lunch, you'll have more energy all day long and you won't be starving later in the day. Do you do something that gets your heart pumping every day? If you don't feel like running or doing an intense workout, just put on some music and dance! Anything that is fun and makes you sweat will help your body be fit, strong and healthy.

Most important, do not start weighing yourself or counting calories. Remember, ED loves numbers. If you start counting things like pounds or calories, it's like inviting ED into your brain. You need to focus on your body and get out of your head. What I mean by that is: eat foods that make you feel good and give you energy. Try to be more active. Listen to and act upon your body's hunger and fullness signals. If you do these things, then you will be healthy, which is more important than being skinny. This way you will be developing habits for having a healthy body for the rest of your life. This is a wonderful gift to give your future you!

Final Wishes

Thanks for visiting! I hope you have a better understanding of body image and the complicated connection between food and feelings. I hope that you can recognize and fight the bully in the brain called ED.

As we say good-bye, I have three wishes for you... and a secret.

- My first wish is that you'll hold onto the important life lessons that you learned here as you move into your teen years.

- My second wish is that you'll continue to explore whatever makes your heart sing and that you'll discover the unique gifts that you have to offer the world.

- My third wish is that you do more than just survive: I hope you thrive. That means that you don't just grow older over the years, but you develop your whole self—mind, body, and spirit—to reach your full potential as a human.

Now for the secret. It's based on the wisdom of the ages. Most people your age do not yet know this secret, but if you really get it, then you'll be well-prepared for a wonderful life. Okay, are you ready?

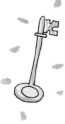

The key to happiness is having positive connections to other people, whether friends or family. Healthy loving relationships are the most important ingredient in recovering from an eating disorder, and they are the best way to fight Ed if he ever dares to show up in the first place. Love beats money, Love beats stuff, Love beats thin.

Always remember, in *Diet Land* all that matters is the number on the scale, the size of your body, and the hopeless quest to be the *Thinnest.* ED's biggest crime is that he steals the gifts of time, attention, and love from this one precious, amazing life that we've been given.

Don't ever let him do it to you!

xo,

Dina